Greater
Vision

Greater Vision

Vision

A Comprehensive Program for Physical, Emotional, and Spiritual Clarity

Marc Grossman, O.D., L.Ac.,
and Vinton McCabe, N.V.E.

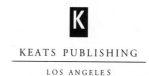

KEATS PUBLISHING

LOS ANGELES

Library of Congress Cataloging-in-Publication Data

Grossman, Marc.
    Greater vision : a comprehensive program for physical, emotional, and spiritual clarity /
Marc Grossman, Vinton McCabe.
       p.   cm.
    Includes bibliographical references and index.
    ISBN 0-658-00643-6
    1. Visual training.   2. Behavioral optometry.   3. Vision disorders—Psychosomatic
aspects.   I. McCabe, Vinton.   II. Title.

RE960.G76   2001
617.7—dc21   00-67784

Keats Publishing

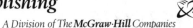

A Division of The McGraw·Hill Companies

1 2 3 4 5 6 7 8 9 0   DOH/DOH   0 9 8 7 6 5 4 3 2 1

ISBN: 0-658-00643-6

This book was set in Janson by Susan H. Hartman
Printed and bound by R. R. Donnelley

Cover design by Hebron Design

McGraw-Hill books are available at special quantity discounts to use as premiums and sales
promotions, or for use in corporate training programs. For more information, please write to
the Director of Special Sales, Professional Publishing, McGraw-Hill, Two Penn Plaza, New
York, NY 10121-2298. Or contact your local bookstore.

This book is printed on acid-free paper.

To my community of friends, whose nourishment I feel every day: Michael Edson, Ellen Marshall, David Lester, Loren Quimby, Bea Ehrsam, Pasquale Strocchia, Mary Goggin, Christina Powers, Paul Barone, Hindy Preskin, Amy Fradon, Hilary Partridge, Zahava Wilson, Diane Nowicki, and Aaron Warshawsky, with special thanks to Carol Douglass for her patience and support while I wrote this book.

To my office staff, who make my work with patients a possibility: Denise Catuogno, Annette Nacinovich, and Lori Sumliner.

To my loving parents, sisters, and their families: Dorothy and Irwin Grossman; Karen, Ronald, Cory, and Jenna Speicher; Lisa, Scott, Steven, and Jessica Ente, and to Tuli.

—Marc Grossman

I would like to thank my patients and coworkers who made my seven years at the Rye Learning Center among the most valuable and exciting of my life.

I would also like to thank Marc Grossman for literally teaching me to see.

And I would like to thank David Dumas. Without his support throughout the long and checkered history of this project, *Greater Vision* would have proved itself to be a mirage.

—Vinton McCabe

Also by Marc Grossman
Natural Eye Care—An Encyclopedia: Complementary Treatments for
   Improving and Saving Your Eyes
Magic Eye: How to See 3D

Also by Vinton McCabe
Homeopathy, Healing, and You
Practical Homeopathy

Contents

SECTION TWO: Exercises for Greater Vision

Foreword

J onathan Swift said that real vision was the ability to see the invisible. *Greater Vision* is about just that, expanding our "seeing" to include what once we could not see. To do that, our insight, not our eyesight, must be healed. We must "see" beyond our beliefs to truly change our vision.

In *Greater Vision*, Marc Grossman and Vinton McCabe not only offer us their knowledge and experiences, but most of all, they share their life's journeys. For one cannot share in such depth what one has not personally experienced.

How often do we deny what we see to avoid discomfort, not recognizing that this conditioned behavior in itself is the cause of our worldwide epidemic of poor eyesight? What would happen if we acknowledged everything we saw, heard, and felt? How would we be different? How would our lives be different?

In the West, we think we see with only two eyes, but in the East they have always been aware of a third eye, "the eye of contemplation," that looks within to see God. When we open our eyes to everything that touches us, we awaken this third eye and experience our deepest inner terrain. In this book, Marc Grossman and Vinton McCabe provide us an invitation and map into this terrain with illuminated signposts. I applaud them for sharing their vision of a new reality.

—Dr. Jacob Liberman, author of
Light: Medicine of the Future,
Take Off Your Glasses and See, *and*
Wisdom from an Empty Mind

Preface

The Amblyope's Revenge

Different cultures would tend to look at my eyes differently. The Italians, for instance, would tend to take one look at my left eye and mutter, "*Malocchio*," before spitting into the dust in front of their feet. The French, who would tend to find my left eye rather lovely, would say that I have been kissed by Aphrodite. In the United States, people tend to say that I have a lazy eye and let it go at that.

Ah, but my eye is so much more than just lazy. I was born with the condition amblyopia. I have a left eye that turns all the way out to the far corner when I am tired or drunk. And more, this left eye is very nearsighted, while my right eye, the one that stares straight ahead of itself as a good eye should, has perfect vision.

There are those who say that people who are born with amblyopia suffer a form of schizophrenia, that their eyes are wired to their brains in a manner that is different from that of the average person. While I would shy away from this particular explanation for my behavior, I do admit that, like a good Italian, I spent a good deal of my life thinking of my left eye as evil and of my right eye, the one that did all the work while the left one wandered about in its socket, as the good eye.

While other people's vision conditions are often overlooked, mine was so apparent to all that it was dealt with in swift order. I was in my first go-round of vision therapy almost as soon as I could walk. And I was wearing glasses by the time I was five.

This is not to say that I did not think that my eyes were functioning just fine on their own. I did. Because my left eye was so nearsighted, it adapted over time to be my close-up eye. I read with it; I did any work with it that required deep concentration. My right eye adapted to be my distance eye. Because its vision was perfect, it could do pretty much anything required of it, but over time it actually became a bit farsighted because of the way in which it was used.

All in all, it seemed to be an excellent adaptation. In fact, I would have recommended it to anyone—having one eye for close-up and one for far away. It seemed to save unnecessary wear and tear of the eyes.

There was only one drawback. I never saw anything with both eyes at the same time. This meant that no matter how many times I put on the red-and-green glasses to do vision therapy work or to try and see a 3-D movie, I would see only red, the color that covered the right eye. Of course, if I was trying to see a 3-D comic book that I held close to my face, then I saw only the green that covered my left eye.

Over time I came to realize that in the first instant of looking at anything, I did use both my eyes—but only for an instant. In that moment, my mind was locking in on which of my eyes would be best used in the circumstance at hand. That eye would, as I came to think of it, come on-line, and the other would drift off into space.

But this drifting led to problems of perception. There were some small ones: It was years before I saw that Superman had an *S* on his chest, for instance. Since I saw the yellow as the dominant color and not the red, I thought on his chest was some Kryptonian symbol. But there were larger ones as well. Most had to do with having an understanding of exactly where I was in relation to everything else. Since I never used both eyes, I had terrible depth perception. Even though the brain, wonderful instrument that it is, has the ability to synthesize depth for those of us who do not see it naturally, this lack of depth perception made everything from dodgeball to driving a car a particular challenge.

And then there is peripheral vision. Since my left eye turns out so far to the side, I have a wide vista-vision effect on that side of my head. Therefore, the world on the right side, where the eye is pretty much nailed in, looks smaller and narrower. To this day, because of this, I am easily startled by anyone or anything that approaches me from the right side. This difference in peripheral vision has, all in all, been the source of greatest visual distortion in my life.

So, I was the perfect candidate for vision therapy, or so it seemed, by the time I was four years old. I wore the patch over my good eye to encourage the lazy one to do some work. I looked at the 3-D cards with the red and green glasses and saw only the red tent. And I stared at the pencil tip with my right eye as it came toward my nose, while my left eye lingered out in the corner like a wallflower at a school dance.

Finally, it was decided that vision therapy was perhaps not for me, and my parents considered surgery. Doctors told them that they could simply cut the muscle that was allowing my eye to wander and stick it back in the center where it belonged. My father thought this was an excellent idea and was immediately ready to sign me up. My mother, however, asked the doctor whether the surgery would actually correct my eyesight or would, instead, be merely cosmetic. When told that my eye would look better but would have no improvement in seeing, she refused to allow the surgery. I remember this time very clearly, although I was very young. I remember the loud arguments between my parents, my father pounding his fist on the kitchen table and my mother refusing to allow the operation to take place.

Finally, with my parents at an angry impasse, I was given a pair of black-rimmed glasses and sent off to the first grade. The doctors found that if the prescription of the left lens was strong enough, not only would it correct my nearsightedness, but it would also pull my eye in so that it would appear normal. My glasses were military issue, a junior pair of the ones that my father always wore.

I remember those glasses very clearly as well. Not because they were a fashion statement, or lack thereof, but because of the pain that they caused. As the doctor put them on my face, I jerked my head back hard to get away. My happy adaptation was gone—no more near eye/far eye. In an instant, the world was changed from a vague blur to distinct images. This was all well and good, but no one had bothered to tell me how much my left eye would hurt when the prescription began to force it into place or how tiring it would be to wear those glasses even for a few minutes. And no one seemed to want to listen when I tried to tell them how poorly the supposed solution was working. But because we were an army family, I had access to almost constant vision care. As often as it was deemed necessary, I was given new, stronger glasses to increase the acuity of my vision and to hold my wandering eye in check.

When I was a teenager, they finally gave me a contact lens for the left eye. As my glasses had had no prescription for the right eye, I didn't need to wear a lens in that eye. I came to consider the contact lens to be a straitjacket for my left eye. But every night when I took the contact out to boil it in its little pot for the next day's wear, my left eye would bounce right out again to the corner of its socket. While it had been strapped in place for a time by the contact lens, nothing about the eye's ability to see had changed.

I know that this will likely sound strange to those whose eyes easily lock on target and whose eyes turn both inward and outward on mental command. But, because of all the pain and strain that treatment caused me, I began to resent my left eye. As a result of all the negative input I got from parents, teachers, and doctors, I came to consider them the good twin and the evil twin. And, although I will still challenge and revile those who would lump amblyopes in with the schizophrenics, I did often wonder why my left eye couldn't at least try to be a bit more like its perfect brother.

It was about thirty years after I first wore glasses that I again gave vision therapy a try. By this time I was seeing a vision specialist who felt that it was wrong for me to wear only one contact lens, even though my right eye saw perfectly. So he fitted me with a lens for the right eye as well and gave me a prescription for that eye that treated it as if it were nearsighted (though it had at one time been considered far-sighted). Now I had straitjackets for both eyes and an increasing problem with migraines as well.

This doctor also gave me contact lenses that I was able to sleep in. At first I truly loved these lenses for that moment each morning when I woke up and opened my eyes. In that moment, I could see clearly through both my eyes. That seemed a miraculous thing to me. And with prescription lenses in front of both my eyes, I could see more clearly than I ever had in my life before. I remember telling my friends that with my contacts I could see through walls.

Over the months, however, I began to understand that this artificial clarity induced by stronger and stronger lenses came at a price. I was getting worse and worse headaches and had an almost constant sense of distortion in my vision. On top of this, I noticed that on that one night every two weeks or so that I had to take the lens out of my left eye and sleep without it, it flew to the corner of the eye like a cowering animal just as soon as the lens was removed. And the quality of my vision in both eyes seemed worse when my lenses were removed.

About this time, I read in Dr. Jacob Liberman's book, *Light: Medicine of the Future*, of a case of a little girl with amblyopia who, after two or three sessions of treatment with light, no longer had a lazy eye. From the back of that book, I got the name and address for a Dr. Marc Grossman, who ran an office called the Rye Learning Center, which supposedly specialized in problems like mine. I called and made my appointment.

My first experience with Marc Grossman was filled with things that I didn't expect. For instance, I didn't expect that the Rye Learning Center would be located in the basement of a condominium complex. Nor did I expect that the rooms of the center would be filled with equipment that looked like it was cast off by the collapsed Soviet Union. And nothing in my previous experience with medical practitioners had told me what to expect from Marc Grossman himself.

There's something about the way that he looks into his patient's eyes. He has a way of actually and totally being in the room with you that can be a bit disconcerting. With extraordinary sensitivity, he seems to bear witness to all that you are and all that you need. He does not look through you or away from you, but directly at you, and you believe that he truly sees you and that he does not in any way judge what he is seeing.

Marc creates a safe space around the two of you. Within that safe and silent place, you find yourself talking not just about your eyes, but about your whole life. And in this first session with Marc, I began to get an understanding that, in his consideration, vision has to do with much more than the eyes. It has to do with the mind and the connection between the mind and the eyes—how well and how effectively the eyes are wired into the brain. Further, vision has to do with the heart, with the emotions, with the wounds in our lives that have not healed properly: emotional scars cause vision blocks. And finally, it has to do with the human spirit; ironically, the part of us that is invisible has the greatest impact on our sense of sight.

After talking with Marc for more than an hour in our first session, I decided that I would give vision therapy another try. During that session, he had dismissed the notion that there was any sort of quick fix for my vision problems and that colored light could be helpful but would not in and of itself solve all my troubles.

So I began what would be a three-year process of vision therapy. Had I known that it would be a three-year process at the outset, it is likely that I would still be wearing two contact lenses and getting migraines today. But, as Marc always does, we began with today and went from there.

I was sent into a small room that looked something like a preschool, with little furniture everywhere. There I was taught my first exercise, Figure 8s. I was to soon learn that the names for the exercises were never figurative. Figure 8s was tracing large figure eights on a wall with your eyes; Turntable was sitting in front of a spinning turntable and trying to trace holes as they spun around and then trying to stick pegs into those holes.

To make things more difficult, I was quickly fitted with therapy glasses. These were glasses that had the opposite prescription to those

I wore in everyday life. Thus I was given a farsighted prescription. I found that I liked these immediately, because they made everything very blurry and I am a fan of blur. I found that I would sigh and relax when I put these glasses on, just as I would unconsciously pull away from the lenses that I wore every day on the street. I also found that, unlike my street glasses these therapy glasses actually improved my vision the more I wore them.

Along these same lines, Marc also got rid of the contact lens in my right eye and lowered the prescription of the lens in my left. He explained to me that the term *prescription* is apt, for glasses and contact lenses are a sort of drug to the system. And like all allopathic drugs, they have side effects. A too-strong prescription could lead to myriad physical and emotional symptoms, including the headaches that I was getting. He could correct all sorts of tension- and stress-related ailments by weakening the prescription in front of my eyes. As is common with him, Marc lowered the potency of the prescription I wore so that while I was still able to see well enough to safely move through the world, I was no longer able to see "through walls." He would continue to lower my prescription throughout my years of therapy as my sight grew naturally stronger and stronger.

And, as is usual for him, Marc gave me a program of home-based exercise, one that he had created specifically for me. I visited the office for a session a week but had exercises that I was to do daily at home.

The first and in many ways most important task of my vision therapy was to awaken my left eye. The vision in it was strong but blurry. So over the years my brain had learned to ignore the information taken in by my left eye.

Because that eye drifted so very far outward, if my brain had not adapted in this manner, I would have had a double image of everything, one that was blurry and one that was clear. So my left eye had become something of an ornament. And now it was time to bring it back on-line.

This was not an easy process. No one had prepared me for just how resistant I would be to change, even though I thought that I had come into vision therapy with every intention of getting well. Nor had anyone prepared me for the fact that there would be physical pain involved in getting that eye moving and in holding it in place. The slightest attempt at convergence, at moving my two eyes together, would bring on physical agony. I can remember leaving those early sessions in a state of emotional and physical exhaustion.

But then, one night, something weird happened. I remember it very clearly. I was watching a rerun of "Knots Landing" on television, and suddenly everything looked completely different. What had always been a relatively flat landscape now had unbelievable depth and clarity. Even the colors looked brighter and sharper. Abby looked incredible.

While it lasted only a moment and I was afraid to blink or move my head, I was actually seeing with both eyes at once. I was thirty-seven years old, and I was finally seeing the way that most people see effortlessly all their lives. The moment was an incredible rush. It was also terrifying. In that instant, the whole world shifted. Nothing looked the way it used to, and nothing was located where it used to be. After a second, everything returned to what I had always considered to be normal. Although I had been really frightened by the experience, I knew that this was what I wanted.

The second time my eyes came on-line together, the experience was not so good. I was driving, having just gotten off of I-95 at my exit, when suddenly everything shifted again, only for a second. But in that second I was moving in space in a way that I had never been aware of moving before. And space was something that was suddenly very deep and very wide. I didn't know how to drive without crashing into something. After a second, everything shifted back again. Only this time, due to the trauma of the event, it would be several months before the left eye would be coaxed back to awareness.

In a case like mine, you never think in terms of welding the eyes back together. You can't try to force fusion. After all, the amblyope's eyes are far more like independent beings than are those of the average person.

The goal of my vision therapy was increased options. Over the years I learned that my original adaptation—near eye/far eye—was, while relatively healthy, one that limited my experience of life. It limited me not only visually but also in terms of who I was and who I could become as a person.

Over the years of my own therapy, the fused state became the more common one for my eyes, but each eye will still move to the dominant position upon occasion. As I write these words, I notice that my left eye is doing the work and my right eye is resting. This is always the case when I do creative work. At tax time, my right eye is dominant.

Vision therapy gave me two things: a sense of understanding of how my eyes worked and how I could come to see and function better in the world, and a better sense of who I am and who I want to be.

Certainly, my vision has improved. My left eye requires a far lower prescription in order to function. And my two eyes work far better as a team, allowing me to see my world as it is and to work dynamically to shape it into what I want it to become.

This last note concerns something that happened only a couple of years ago, years after I had ended my own vision therapy and had begun practicing as a vision therapist myself and more than a decade after the death of my father.

I remember my last look at my father, laid out in his coffin, still wearing those black-rimmed army glasses. In the seventies, I had begun to wear aviators; in the eighties, I went with those huge, square, plastic frames that I called my Elton John glasses; and in the nineties, I discovered BADA and Occuli Armani. But my father stayed strictly with his military issue, even after he retired from thirty years of service.

Years after his funeral, I was talking with my mother on the phone, telling her about what I had learned about myself and my own personal vision through the process of my vision therapy. After a pause in the conversation, my mother said, "It's a pity that your father didn't live long enough to hear all this." While it certainly was a pity that my father was no longer alive, I didn't understand why it was a pity that he could not hear about this specifically and said so.

"Well, because," my mother said. "His eyes were just like yours. I mean, his left eye was just like yours. Didn't you ever notice how thick his left lens was in his glasses? That's why he always wore those plastic frames—because the lens didn't show so much. But his left eye turned out just like yours. That's why he got so upset when you were born and he saw your eye. He felt like he had given you a disease, that you had inherited his weakness. When he was little, he didn't have glasses. It was during the Great Depression, after all. So the other kids tormented him about his eye turning out. That's why he wanted you to have the operation so badly, and why you got glasses so young, and why he never would let you take them off. Because then he would have to see your eye turn."

Thinking about it afterward, I realized that I had never seen my father without his glasses. He literally wore them all the time. They seemed to have been a physical part of his face. And it seemed so odd, all these years later, that something that we actually had in common should stand between us in a very real way. What he had seen as a weakness, a taint, I had always seen as a special gift, a talent in a way. My left eye made me different, yes, but it also made me special, in the same way that my friends who were double-jointed seemed special. It was a trick, like curling your tongue or wiggling your ears. I not only didn't mind other people seeing my eye without the glasses that held it in place, I rather forced it on them by forever taking my glasses off and forgetting where I'd put them. Where my father saw his glasses as something that could make him appear normal—although he considered himself to be abnormal because of the curse of his evil eye—I equated my glasses with restriction and pain. To this day I enjoy taking them off and losing them. I drop them with the same fervor that the crippled drop their crutches onstage at revival meetings, with a sense of freedom and joy.

So this ends with the missed opportunity: my not being able to thank my father for the legacy he thought so terrible and show him that I can bring my eyes together or let them wander when I choose. I wish I could have offered him the same freedom that I myself have found.

                                                              —*Vinton McCabe*

Acknowledgments

This book would not have been possible without the support of many different people. The authors would like to thank the following for the permission to use their materials as part of this book: Sam Berne, O.D.; Roberto Kaplan, O.D.; Fredrick Franck; Jason Elias, L.Ac.; Gary Zukav; Paul Harris, O.D.; Michael Samuels, M.D.; Baxter Swartwout, O.D.; and especially the Optometric Extension Program for all its work and materials dedicated to the concept of behavioral vision care.

I am indebted to many people and organizations that have supported me on my path in my work with vision. I would like to thank my teachers, colleagues, patients, and friends who through the years gave me the confidence and support to go beyond the traditional way of looking at vision care.

To my optometric family whose work has inspired me: Drs. Sam Berne, Ray Gottlieb, Roberto Michael Kaplan, Jacob Liberman, Albert Sutton, Abe Shapiro, Larry Wallace, Paul Harris and the Vermont Study Group, and others too numerous to mention, with special gratitude to my two primary mentors, Drs. Albert Shankman and Elliot Forrest.

To the following organizations that go beyond the traditional way of looking at life and healing and that gave me the confidence to explore new ways of looking at vision: The Optometric Extension Program, whose work over the last seventy years was the foundation for many of the concepts in this book; Omega Institute and Dance New England, who help supply a safe environment for me to be innovative in my work with vision.

To other colleagues in the healing professions who have been generous to me in sharing their views of vision so that I may learn more: Drs. Catherine Sweet and Ron Wish, with special thanks to my friend, mentor, and partner at Integral Health Associates, Jason Elias, for his inspiration and help.

To our editor, Peter Hoffman, at Keats Publishing, for being so cooperative and supportive in the publishing of this book.

To my patients over the last twenty years, who gave me the opportunity to really begin to understand the meaning of having greater vision.

—*Marc Grossman*

Introduction

Put yourself in my place for a moment. Someone that you have never seen before has come into your office and is sitting in your chair. You've taken a moment before she came in to go over the forms that she filled out while she sat in the waiting room. They tell you mostly about expectations—what she expects of you. Something has brought her into your office. You look over the checklist of symptoms: itching eyes, sleepiness upon reading, photophobia, and the like. And then you watch her walk across the floor of your office. You can tell a lot about her just by the way she moves, the strength of her grip as she takes your hand. And then she sits in the chair and looks up, expectant.

And you look directly into her eyes.

I am often asked what I see when I look into a patient's eyes. I used to say that before I could make that intimate connection with another person, I had to first be sure that I myself was centered and ready. I had to first be sure of where I was and how I was feeling. If I was feeling distracted and not present in the room with this other person, I had to first make myself willing to be this person's witness, his or her mirror.

I used to say that when I looked into my patients' eyes, I first saw their emotional state, their anxiousness, their fear. And then I would see the aspects of their mind, their presence. I would discern their pilot light, if you will—whether their personal energy was dulled or active, whether they turned to flight or fight in times of stress.

But there's more to it.

The eyes are, after all, simply tools of the mind. They are made out of brain tissue, as if the brain itself has pushed its way out of the skull, in the same way and for the same reason that a seed pushes its way out of the soil: in order to see the light. The eyes are the brain's expression of itself on the surface of the human body, the method by which the brain knows the world and gathers enough information to make itself known to the world at large. To me, that is why the eyes are so mysterious, so filled with meaning. These tools (basically they are just video cameras mounted on the front of our heads) allow us to interrelate our minds with the world around us. Without them, so much would be lost: so much knowledge, so much understanding, and so much mystery.

And yet, I can't truly say that the eyes are simply receptive in their function. They are organs of both giving and receiving. They are reflections of our soul, of who and where we are at any given moment on all levels of being—physical, emotional, mental, and spiritual.

On a sense level, the first place that people block out information is with their eyes. When stress of any sort becomes too great, when people no longer feel that they can safely deal with the world, they may close down their visual system. Some will do this by becoming nearsighted, by living in an ongoing state of blur. Others will close off their peripheral vision in an attempt to close off the immensity of the world.

Intellectually, we begin our lives as a tabula rasa. As newborns we see through eyes that are clear and searching. As we develop, we learn from our parents, our schools, and our own experience. Our mind interweaves with our emotions. Information that has been recorded visually, through the link between the mind and the eyes, is recorded within a context that involves our intellect and our emotions. If a scary-looking man was mean to me, then when next I see a scary-looking man, I will place that man within the context of things to avoid, and I will take the action appropriate to that context, whether or not it is based in the reality of the situation. In the same way, intellect and emotions become intertwined with experiences involving environment, circumstances, and actions. If I almost drown the first time I swim, I may need only to see water in any form to bring about a physical, mental, and emotional response within my being.

Edward Whitmont, a Jungian analyst and homeopath, has said that that which cannot be digested on an emotional level will make us physically ill. And this concept is borne out in our visual system. If we have seen something that causes us stress and if we cannot work through the context of that vision to understand and learn from it, then we might well develop a physical vision impairment. That our emotional state impacts the quality of our vision is true without a doubt. We all experience this as in the course of every day we have moments when things seem dull and rather blurry and moments of exciting clarity. Those of us who are placed in situations in which stress is ongoing or who have received a shock sufficient to cause long-lasting effects may well develop chronic complaints. In my practice I have seen many dozens of patients who have suddenly and seemingly without reason or cause developed problems with their vision after their families have been rocked by divorce or by the death of a loved one. I have also seen patients who develop vision troubles after losing their jobs or after career setbacks.

And there is a spiritual component to vision as well. Having spent the better part of twenty years in the study and practice of behavioral optometry, I cannot help but conclude that our problems with our visual sense—our lack of vision, if you will—are what keep us from living in a state of grace. That state is one in which we are in harmony with ourselves and others.

In that state of grace we are experiencing dynamic freedom as well: to live as we truly are and as we want to be, and to enjoy the abundance that life offers us without fear, denial, or the burdens placed upon us by grief. When we are in this state of grace, we live in the present moment. We are aware—truly aware—of all that is taking place around us. It is that almost magical flow in which we do not trip over our own two feet.

I believe that this state of grace will always carry with it a sense of greater vision and that a sense of greater vision will lead us to a state of grace.

We have all heard the adage that for lack of a vision the cause is lost. In this simple phrase, we have the two distinct meanings of the word *vision* intertwined. The phrase refers both to the inability to see something clearly and to the inability to understand it, because the two are irrevocably bound together. They are, in fact, the same thing.

Remember: the eyes are in part actually formed from brain tissue. The reality is that our organs of sight do more than simply see. Our ability to see is irrevocably linked with our ability to understand, grow, and change.

As we move through our lives, all of us encounter catalyst after catalyst, each of which elicits a response of some sort from within us. The catalyst may be a car that nearly cuts us off as we drive or a beautiful sunrise, but our lives are populated with events that cause us to react in some way—physically, emotionally, mentally, or spiritually. These responses may be balanced and healthy or reckless and foolish, but they largely determine both our sense of sight and our personal vision. At worst, these responses may become a pattern of destruction, which leads us toward ill health on all levels of being. But at best, as our responses to specific catalysts change over the years, as we learn which of our decisions were wise and which were foolish, we undergo the process of *personal evolution*. It is the purpose of this book to be a guide for creative change and personal evolution, so that through an understanding of the complexities of the visual system, you may find yourself on a path of increased clarity.

But *Greater Vision* can offer something more. It can offer a personal transformation, which is the ability to make the changes necessary in your life not slowly and over time, but in an instant of clarity and understanding.

To do this, we must first change our goals. When dealing with our eyes, we have until now set forth the goal of *better* vision. By this I mean we seek acuity, clarity of sight. We want to read the chart across the room so that our eye doctor will tell us that we don't need stronger glasses.

But the goal of *Greater Vision* is so much more than this. To really work on clarity of vision, you must work on yourself as a whole being and you must come to understand that vision involves relationships.

Even on the most basic level, sight involves the intimate relationship between the person seeing and the object or person being seen. On a more profound level, vision evolves based upon your relationships with yourself, your loved ones, your community, your world, and your God. Therefore, your ultimate goal should never stop with simple visual clarity. Rather, it is that you should attain spiritual clarity.

Better vision is the domain of the eye care professional who selects for you the most efficient pair of contact lenses or glasses. For her, your sight is a matter of the eyeball, the retina, and the brain. This doctor, while making her selection, will ask you which is better as she changes the lenses in front of your eyes. This doctor will ask which is better in terms of clarity alone, never which of the two feels better. And yet your feelings determine the quality of your sight every bit as much as your retinas do.

If we are to experience greater vision, we must start by knowing who we are and where we are in relation to the world. We must learn our role and place. And we must bring into harmony the objective reality of the world with our own very personal, subjective form of reality. The closer the two match, the more clearly we are in harmony with all that surrounds us and the more easily we may move through our lives. Our reality may be clouded by so many things—emotions like fear and hate, lack of mental clarity, and chronic physical complaints— all of which we have to learn to transcend if we are finally to be free.

Certainly the prospect of greater vision encompasses better vision. If we are to see clearly and well with our spirits, we must also see clearly and efficiently with our physical eyes. By *efficiently*, I mean that we must, even on the physical level, transcend our lust for simple acuity. We must learn to balance our physical vision with all its components.

Therefore, this is a book about relationships and change—about our ability to grow, on every level of being.

To go back to the question that opened these pages, I am asked what I see when I look into a patient's eyes.

To answer this I must first point out that traditional Chinese medicine stresses that the health of our beings is determined by the health of our meridians. These *meridians* are pathways of energy that flow through our beings, through our bodies, minds, and spirits. When there are inefficiencies in these pathways, blocks of the free flow of the energy, disease is created on one or more levels of our being.

It has always been deeply meaningful to me that every single one of these meridians goes through the eyes. All of our energy, all that we are, flows through them. This energy not only flows through the eyes but travels from there to the human heart. The link between our minds and our hearts expresses the sum of who we are.

It is possible, therefore, that when I look into a patient's eyes, I can see all that there is to see about that human, if only I know how to see it and to understand it.

Again, the Chinese have a word for it. They say that your eyes hold your *shen*, which is the word for "spirit." When I look into your eyes, that is what I see first, your *shen*, your spirit, your perfect white light.

Understanding Greater Vision

CHAPTER 1

Sight

Discovering the Image

"Use the light that is within you to regain your natural clearness of sight. Seeing into darkness is clarity. Knowing how to yield is strength. Use your own life and return to the source of light. This is called practicing eternity."

—Lao-tze

The function of the eye as an organ is to create an image in your mind. But to understand what this means and how this vital process works, you must first understand the difference between sight and vision.

Sight occurs on a physical level of being that includes the retina, the eyeball, the lens, and the other physical parts of the eye. It involves *acuity*, the clarity of the image seen. On the level of pure sight, comprehension of the image is not important. We do not need to understand what we have seen; we only need to see it clearly.

Vision, on the other hand, takes place within the mind and spirit, as well as within our physical bodies. And vision involves more than simple clarity of the image seen. It involves our ability to interpret the image that we see, and it is how we use what we have seen. Comprehension, therefore, may be said to be the key to our sense of vision. And the greater our ability to comprehend, interpret, and use what we take in visually, the greater our sense of personal vision.

3

This is not to say that sight itself is not important. Certainly if we have a problem with the sensory input—which is what sight is—if the image received is not clear, then we might experience both mental and physical stress in attempting to see, understand, and make use of the information that we have seen.

Therefore, before you make use of the vision we have and broaden and deepen it into a sense of greater vision, you must learn to understand the process of sight. If the mechanical parts of the eye are working efficiently, you have optimal potential for greater vision.

A Map of the Human Eye

As author Bethany Argixle puts it, "Eyes are delicate, transparent, ever-changing with what they reflect. Eyes reach out and they take in. The eye receives the image."

The human eye is everything that Argixle states that it is. As an object of beauty and mystery it is without parallel in all creation. It is

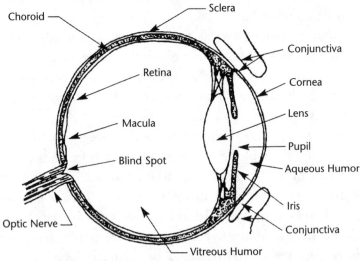

Reprinted with permission from *Smart Medicine for Your Eyes* by Jeffrey Anshel. New York: Avery Publishing, 1999.

perhaps for this reason that ancient cultures selected their most precious and valuable gems to represent the eyes in their statues. No other sense organ so connects us with the universe around us or so deeply represents us in our desire to understand that universe as does the eye. Unlike our other sense organs, the human eye is partially structured from brain tissue. Just as sunlight nurtures and sustains life on our planet, light powers our sense of vision, opening our minds to an unending vista of color, shape, and, most important, meaning.

But to understand vision and meaning, you must first understand sight. To understand sight, you must first learn the basic structure involved in seeing.

The *orbit* is the space in the skull in which the eye is located. The eyeball, the optic nerve, the eye muscles, and the nerves of the eye are all found within the orbit.

The *eyelids*, located on the outside of the eye and on top of and below the orbit, protect the eye from injury and from excessive light. They also help keep the cornea moist.

The *eyeball* itself is contained within the center of the orbit. It is only two and a half centimeters in length and is attached to a series of six muscles, which move the eyeball in all directions. These are called the *extraocular muscles*. A series of three cranial nerves supply innervation to the eye via the six extraocular muscles.

The *conjunctiva* of the eye is a thin, clear membrane that covers the white of the eye, which is called the *sclera*.

The white tissue of the sclera is an external coat covering five-sixths of the eye. The other one-sixth of the eye is the transparent structure called the *cornea*. The cornea is an extremely important structure of the eye because it is the key optical component responsible for the refraction of light that enters the eye. It is an unusual tissue in the human body because it is clear and has no blood vessels.

Directly behind the cornea is a clear, watery fluid called the *aqueous humor*, which fills the anterior chamber of the eye.

Next after the aqueous humor is the *lens* of the eye, a flexible structure that, like the cornea, is transparent and has no blood vessels and is another key part of the refractive system of the eye. The lens is important for the process of accommodation, for focusing the image so that it is seen clearly. The lens does not do this by changing its position in the eye but by changing its shape. The lens is actually not completely solid, but is built up of thin layers, like an onion. The lens capsule is a clear, membranelike structure that is very elastic—a quality that allows it to remain in a state of constant tension.

When the *ciliary muscle* relaxes, the ciliary processes pull on the suspensory ligaments, which, in turn, pull the lens capsule around its equator. This causes the entire lens to flatten, or become less convex. This enables the lens to focus light from objects at a distance. Likewise, when the ciliary muscle contracts, tension is released on the supensory ligaments and on the lens capsule, causing both lens surfaces to become more convex again, allowing the eye to refocus on objects up close. This adjustment in lens shape in order to focus at various distances is referred to as *accommodation*. To summarize the process, the flatter the lens, the better we can see at a distance, and the fatter the lens, the better we can see close-up. The lens is normally fat when the ciliary muscle is contracted and flat when the muscle is relaxed.

It is within the lens that many of our vision troubles develop as we age. The lens is built and rebuilt constantly throughout our lives, and new cells are added as needed. These cells are added from the center outward, making the cells in the direct center of the lens the oldest cells in that part of the eye. These center cells, being the oldest and the cells farthest from the blood system that brings oxygen and nutrients to the eye, die off. When they die, they harden, so that the lens becomes too stiff to change shape as needed, making it harder and harder for the eye to effectively see close-up or at a distance. This is why many middle-aged people suddenly find that they are holding the newspaper at arm's length in order to read it. And also, when too many cells die and clump together, they ultimately will form an opaque section in the lens, which is called a *cataract*.

Behind the lens is where the *vitreous humor* is found. This is a transparent, jellylike substance that contains a meshwork of collagen fibers. It consists of 99 percent water and forms four-fifths of the eye-ball. In addition to transmitting light, it holds the retina in place and provides support for the lens.

At this point I must return to the front of the eyeball itself for a moment to discuss the final structure contained in the eye, the *eyeball*. The eyeball has three concentric coats.

The outermost coat is the sclera, which has been previously discussed.

The middle coat contains the iris, the ciliary body, and the choroid. The *iris* is the colored part of the eye that is located between the cornea and the lens. Eye color depends on the amount and distribution of pigment within the iris. In the middle of the iris is a circular hole that changes in size as the iris muscles expand and contract in response to light. This black hole is called the *pupil*. It acts like an aperture on a camera. The size of the iris changes to regulate the amount of light entering the eye through the pupil. The *ciliary body* lies between the iris and the choroid. Its role is to secrete aqueous humor. It also contains the ciliary muscle, which control the focusing of the lens of the eye. The *choroid* is a dark brown membrane that extends from the ciliary body and covers the entire back of the eye. The choroid contains the blood vessels needed for nutrition of the retina.

The most internal coat of the eye is the *retina*, which is a very thin, delicate membrane. The term *retina* means "net" or "cobweb" and relates to the appearance of blood vessels within the retina. The retina has two layers: an outer pigment cell layer and an internal neural layer. In the back of the retina is a circular depressed area called the *optic disc*. This is where the optic nerve enters the eye and where its fibers spread out in the neural layer of the eye. Because the optic disk has only nerve fibers in it and no photoreceptor cells (rods or cones), it is insensitive to light. This is the part of the eye responsible for creating the blind spot that we notice most often when we drive.

The rods and the cones are light receptors. They are named for the simple geometric shape they resemble when seen under a microscope. *Cones* are found in the central part of the retina, the area in which they receive the brightest light. This is important because it means cones can function only when in fully lighted conditions. When functioning properly, they give us our ability to see details—most important, perhaps, to see colors. In the human eye, the number of cones is about the same as the number of people in New York City.

The *rods* are located in the periphery of the retina. Here they receive less direct light, which is important to their function because it means that they discern no specific colors, only shades of gray. They also discern images far less clearly than do the cones. Rods cannot see objects better than 20/400 which is the size of the largest *E* on the eye chart. Rods deal with peripheral vision and with the ability to detect motion. There are about 130 million rods in the human eye.

Another very important spot on the retina just lateral to the optic disc is the *macula*, in the center of which is an area called the *fovea*. This is the spot where the most precise detail vision is created. It allows us to see clearly and with the greatest detail.

In looking at the retina from its center to its periphery, it might be said that we travel back in evolutionary time, from the most highly organized structure to a "primitive" eye that does little more than detect shadows and movement. In fact, the far periphery of the retina does not even truly respond to movement. Instead, it initiates a reflex for us to direct our eyes to the source of movement so that we can see it with our foveal, or "evolved" eye.

The reflex that directs movement from the periphery to the center of the eye is key to our sense of sight. When we look at an object we align our eyes so that the light from the object is focused onto the fovea of both eyes. This looking involves movement of the eyes. Our eyes are in a constant state of movement, and they move in various ways. When we move our eyes about while searching for a target, we move them quite differently than we do when tracking a target. These eye movements, called *pursuit* eye movements (the process by which the eyes smoothly move to track a target) and *saccadic* eye movements (from the French for "flick of a sail," eye movements in a series of small, rapid jerks while searching for a target), are used to keep the light focused on the fovea of each eye. In this way, when we target our eyes on an object, whether still or in motion, we see it as clearly, precisely, and fully as possible, with (thanks to the two eyes in our targeting system) depth and a full range of color.

The Visual Pathway (An Overview)

Generally, we each come equipped with two eyes and one head. Because the two eyes are located in different positions in the head, each takes a unique view from its own perspective. With these two different, side-by-side perspectives, we are actually able to see a little bit around solid objects without moving our head. So, while the view for each of the two eyes has a good deal in common, each eye captures its own view of reality and separately sends that information to the brain for processing.

This information travels to the brain via the *optic nerve*, which is the main "trunk line," consisting of a million or so separate nerve fibers. It conducts nervous impulses from the retina to the brain.

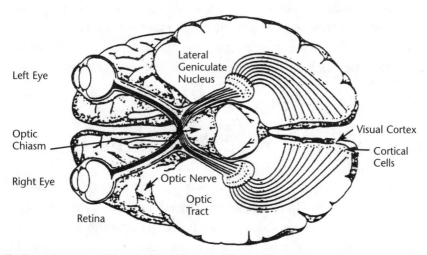

The Eyes as Extensions of the Brain. Illustration by Bunji Tagawa. Reprinted with permission of the estate of Bunji Tagawa.

These impulses send the image taken in by the eye from the eye to the brain. The optic nerve exits from the back of the eyeball and then joins with the optic nerve of the other eye in the area called the *optic chiasm*. From here, the impulses end up in the occipital cortex in the rear of the brain, where the components of the image—color, relative size of objects, motion, and distance—are analyzed.

When the two images arrive simultaneously in the back of the brain, they unite in one picture. The brain combines the two images by matching up the similarities—the areas of the image common to the picture presented by each eye—and then adds the small differences that each eye offers to the overall picture. And although these differences may seem minor, they add up to a major difference to the image itself. Because of the combined information that is common to both eyes and the information unique to each, the completed image is fully three-dimensional, with a perception of depth as well as of color and detail.

This depth perception, called *stereo vision*, most likely evolved as a means of human survival. With stereo vision, we can see where objects are located with much greater precision, especially when those objects are in movement toward or away from us. And because stereo vision helps us to perceive the small difference in the image presented to the brain, it is our best tool for decoding visual camouflage. Thanks to stereo vision, our ancestors could spot the lion hiding in the brush or the poisonous snake coiled in the tree, allowing in part for the survival of the human race. Today, we still depend upon stereo vision for our survival every time we catch a ball, swat a mosquito, or, especially, drive a car.

Light: The Power Behind the Image

Our eyes need light. To be healthy, they need the light of the sun. Light energy reaches the retina and is then transmitted to the brain so that we can see. Light is the force that powers vision.

And yet, the rods and cones within the human eye "see" less than 1 percent of the sun's total electromagnetic spectrum. About 80 percent of the sun's radiation that penetrates our atmosphere is made up of the part of the electromagnetic spectrum known as visible light.

Within the spectrum of visible light, in bright sunlight the human eye is most sensitive to yellow-green light and least sensitive to violet and red light. In darkness, the human eye is most sensitive to green light.

The light that enters through the eyes is used by the body in two distinct ways: first, as mentioned above, light travels into the visual cortex of the brain, where it forms a coherent picture of the world seen; second, light energy also travels to the hypothalamus, which then sends messages to the pineal and pituitary glands based on the information carried by the light energy. The pineal and pituitary glands then send messages throughout the system to regulate many of the functions of the body.

The hypothalamus is often called the master gland of the human body because it functions rather like the operating system of a computer, overseeing the function of the whole system. The hypothalamus itself is very dependent upon both the quality and quantity of the light it receives from the eyes. For example, the hypothalamus regulates the pineal gland, which itself secretes the substance melatonin at night to relax the body and prepare it for sleep. And low light is required in order for the hypothalamus to send the signal to the pineal gland to begin the flow of melatonin. Bright light will inhibit the pineal gland in its function. That is why something as simple as too bright a lamp by the bedside can create insomnia. The pineal gland oversees our "body clock," taking in messages from the hypothalamus on when to begin and end the sleep cycle and sending messages back to the hypothalamus so that it can regulate other body functions within this cycle.

The hypothalamus, working in concert with the pineal and pituitary glands, regulates and oversees such essential functions as sleeping, eating, energy level, growth, body temperature, and blood pressure. And the energy source that powers all of this is light.

A Brief History of Optics

"The nature of sight and the structure of the organ of vision rank among the foremost subjects with which the minds of thinking men have been preoccupied since the dawn of recorded history," wrote S. L. Polyak in his 1941 work *The Retina*, and it is as true today as when he wrote it. Its truth, in fact, has been displayed for over two millenia.

It was Galen, the Greek physician working in Rome in the second century A.D. who, having been inspired by the Greek philosopher Plato before him, stated that he believed that a "visual spirit"—a *pneuma* in his terminology—existed in the human brain and traveled from the brain along the hollows of the optic nerve to the crystalline lens of the eye. There it met the rays of light coming to it from all the objects in the environment. This pneuma then would again travel along the optic nerve and return to the brain, bringing with it the visual image of what it had seen.

By simply substituting *retina* for *pneuma*, you can see that even the ancients had a strong grasp of the visual process. The most interesting part of Galen's theory is perhaps the fact that he felt that the eye was a sending as well as a receiving organ. Galen's theory maintained that the pneuma, as it reached the lens, would send rays into the world as well as take in the light rays emitted by the world around it. This concept of an interplay between the eye and its external environment, this exchange of "rays," has been shown to be true in modern vision research, although exactly what the interchange involves and how it takes place has not yet been determined.

The great genius Leonardo da Vinci theorized that rays of light form an image on the "frontal end of the optic nerve." But Leonardo was troubled by the necessity of an erect image within the eye. Because his own experiments with optics produced an inverted image, as seen within a lens, Leonardo conceived that there are two successive images in the eye: the first obtained from the pupil acting as an aperture in a camera and therefore inverted from the original, external image; the second restored to normal by refraction through the crystalline lens.

By the mid–sixteenth century, science got nearer the truth when Maurolycus theorized that rays of light from an external point enter the eye and are there collected on one point within the retina by the process of refraction through the lens. It was Maurolycus who first believed that the retina was the site of light reception within the eye.

In the 1600s Johannes Kepler insisted that it is the cornea that is mainly responsible for the bending of light rays within the eye and that the lens had a role—due to its ability to change shape—in helping to focus the image on the retina. As for the then-ongoing debate as to what happens to the original, inverted image in the eye and brain, Kepler said that this turning of the inverted image back to right side up was due to the "activity of the Soul." By this he meant that it is a psychological process and not a physiological one. And in this answer he has been proven correct.

By the beginning of the nineteenth century, scientists were becoming more interested in the nature of light. In 1800, an obscure scientist known only as Herschel found that a portion of the sun's radiation extended beyond the spectrum of visible light. The discovery of electromagnetism in 1865 and the x-ray in 1895 proved that visible light is only a small fraction of the sun's total radiation.

Visual Development

To this point, I have discussed the physical parts of the human eye, but the development of that eye and of the sense of sight is also of great importance. Take a moment to consider how a child's sense of sight develops in the first years of life, from the time he leaves the womb until the time he leaves the home and enters the adult world of school.

There are perhaps no more beautiful eyes than the eyes of an infant. These are eyes that act the part of searchlights as they scan and sweep their way across what is literally, for them, a new world.

The eyes are so important to that infant's development and survival that they are already preparing for the tasks that lie ahead of them while that infant is still in the womb. The eyes of the fetus begin to move when the fetus is in its third month of development. The eyes are practicing the movements that will be necessary for them to be able to examine their world when the child is born. And the practice will continue through birth because of the importance of the task. The ability for the infant to actively examine his world is so connected to his growth and development that without proper visual scanning skills, normal development can either slow or stop entirely.

In his first two weeks of life, the infant will establish that his own body is a solid object. From this understanding, he will begin to orient himself in relation to other solid objects and within the realm of physical space. Watch how hard a newborn works. When you lift a baby, notice that his eyes and body move in coordination with each other; eye motion leads to body motion. Unlike the adult, who is well aware of the relation of objects in physical space, the infant is learning, reaching, first with his eyes and then with his hands.

While the infant is in this first, vital stage of development, he needs stimulation in the form of light for normal growth to occur. He needs not only different forms of light but also different patterns of light and shadow as well. Studies have shown that if the infant's visual system is not stimulated by light, normal development is retarded or stopped.

Up until the second month of the child's life, his eyes can focus to a distance of eight to ten inches, or about the arm's length that separates the child's eyes from his mother's when he is being held. Research has shown that a child's attention is usually focused on his mother's mouth until he is three months of age. At that time, development in the cerebral cortex steers that focus to his mother's eyes. This eye-to-eye contact between parent and child has been proven to be vital to the overall development of the child. The loving interplay between parent and child builds the child's ability to lovingly bond with others throughout his whole life.

During these first three months, the baby moves through a stage of development that is oral and passive. He is dependent upon his mother for food and comfort. He learns the oral processes of sucking and eating. And as his oral needs are met, he learns to trust his mother as provider and to feel safe and comfortable in his environment. It is important to note that if the child's needs are not met at this stage, the child will develop a deep distrust with his environment, which can lead to both emotional and visual issues in the future.

The child's development during the first three months, therefore, lays the basis for that child's lifelong ability to establish and maintain contact with the world.

By the end of the third month of life, the infant's visual system also begins to retain all the information that it receives. Until this time, the eyes have, as I have stated above, been searchlights, shining out into all the world and seeking as much visual information as possible. But this information is processed without judgment or context. What is seen is simply seen. But by the third month, other developments have taken place in the child's body that impact visual skills.

By this time, the sheath of fatty tissue called *myelin* that surrounds the nerves of the body has grown and extended to reach the nerves that enter the cerebral cortex. This myelin sheathing helps the nerves to send their visual messages to the brain. But at the time of birth, the infant's myelin sheathing extended only along the optic nerve to the lower part of the brain. Now the sheathing extends into the higher centers of the brain—the parts of the brain that are responsible for more intellectual judgments about what is being seen and how that fits into the context of the whole. By the end of the third month of life, brain wave signals that occur only when visual information is being actively studied can be detected in the baby's brain.

At four months of age, the child begins to develop the ability to consciously control the movements of his eyes. He also learns to coordinate the movements of his eyes with his arms so that he can directly interact with solid objects, starting a hands-on process of learning.

This is the start of what is called *object permanence*, the ability of the child to recognize objects for being what they are. The child also learns specific aspects of objects, whether they are hard or soft, round or square—all the aspects that are necessary for the development of language.

At this age, the child will also begin to develop eye-teaming skills—the working of the two eyes together to target one specific object—which will allow for stereo vision. Once the child's two eyes begin to work together, the child will be able to locate where an object is in relation both to other objects in space and to himself. The development of stereo vision (also called *binocularity*) is the basis from which the child will begin to really and concretely explore his environment. It allows for the child to develop a true sense of space and the ability to track objects as he moves through that space.

With the development of the concept of space, the child will also begin to develop a sense of his own personal space, which most often extends an arm's length around him. Objects that enter the child's personal space will be of great interest to him, as they have entered into an arena of his direct control. Once the concept of personal space is established and recognized as a small part of the overall environment, the child begins to develop an interest in taking his portable, personal space into the world around him.

The child begins crawling during the period of four to eight months of age. The child's focus increases from arm's length to as far as three feet away. With his new mobility, the child continues to develop his ability to see distances as he becomes more and more aware of the environment around him.

At six months of age, the baby begins to use his two eyes together to target objects so that he can grasp them and bring them to him. He begins to gather more and more objects into his personal space. He will also tend at this stage to put objects into his mouth as he studies them. At this point, the child's personal space begins to enlarge as well, from the original eight inches to an average of a full foot.

At nine months, the child begins to explore the environment from a new, vertical perspective through standing. By this point, the child's eyes and hands have formed a full partnership with which he can explore a three-dimensional world. By the tenth month, the child has learned to fully grasp objects, although he is not nearly as skilled at releasing them. His emotional development may mirror his physical development, as the child may be skilled at engaging new things but may have trouble disengaging. The flow of ability to engage and then disengage tends to fully develop around the fourteenth month.

It is during the time period of six months to one year that perhaps the most profound development occurs: the child begins to conceive of himself as an individual who is separate from the world around him.

By the end of the first year of life, the child's visual sense develops a level of comprehension. Now the baby begins to imitate others as they do things. For example, he will stick out his tongue as his caregiver does and imitate other facial expressions. At this level of development, the child's environment extends to ten feet. Within this area, the child will notice objects and persons, make eye contact, and socialize with others. Now the child begins to make a show of his independence in his world. He explores everything: objects, rooms, containers of all sorts. He makes marks on paper. He builds with blocks. He makes contact with others.

By the end of the next year of his life, the child has become sophisticated enough that his eye movements are no longer connected to body motions. That is, he is able to do things with his hands without the direct guidance of his eyes.

As the child develops further, his eyes can begin to coordinate with his entire body, as they once did with his hands. He can now begin to move through space, as the newly developed sense of visual memory—an understanding of the environment based upon past experience of it—guides that motion.

By the second half of the second year, the child has fully developed all visual skills at an arm's length. And his eye-hand skills have developed to the point that he can draw things that he has seen as well as draw vertical and horizontal lines. Further, he is now able to focus on the quantities of things (although the direct concept of numbers has yet to be developed) and the categories into which those things can be placed.

Between ages three and four, the child develops the ability to coordinate the two sides of his body. This will further enhance his eyes' ability to work as a team. And the better the eyes work as a team, the more the child will know the precise location of objects in the environment. During this period, the child also becomes much more social, as his environment enlarges beyond ten feet. Perhaps the most important development at this age has to do with the beginnings of imagination. Where once the child's sense of sight was strictly literal and nonjudgmental, now he begins to visualize as well as see. The child's play begins to include fantasy, and he is able to visualize a world beyond his immediate reality.

At this point, the child is able to successfully complete tasks and develop plans, again based in visual memory, that allow him to carry the tasks to completion.

By age four, through his skills at visualization, the child has developed the ability to be aware of two sides to a situation. This is the beginning for the development of empathy skills. Now the child can visualize himself in someone else's position, see the world from another person's point of view. Physically, the child's ability to integrate the two sides of his body greatly improves at this stage.

By five years of age, the child's visual acuity has reached the point at which he can interact with objects up to twenty feet away and maintain eye contact within that space. At this stage, the child feels that he is able to enter into the adult world. He is ready to leave home and go to school.

When the child enters school, he must be able to see clearly in order to learn. Further, he must be able to control his body in order to sit still and pay attention in class. While this seems simple, it involves an integration between the child's balance mechanism and his visual attention mechanism. He also needs to be able to monitor what is going on in his environment, which takes good eye movement skills. He has to use his pursuit eye movement skills in order keep his attention on the moving target of the teacher in the front of the room. He will also need to develop saccadic eye movement skills in order to move his eyes from target to target in the classroom.

In that classroom, the child makes use of the same visual skills that he will need to call upon throughout his life to move within his ever-enlarging world, to recognize what he is seeing, and to make use of the memory of what he has seen in order to successfully perform his life's tasks.

Primary Visual Skills

Finally, having now considered the mechanics of the eye and the development of the sense of sight, let us consider for a moment the components of that sense and what skills are necessary for us to be able to say that we are seeing things correctly. Consider what an eye care professional sees as he conducts a routine eye exam.

Start with reading an eye chart. With this simple test, the examiner can test three important skills: sight, acuity, and vision.

1. **Sight** is measured by the response of the eye to any light that enters it. The eye will move to align itself with any light source in order to gain the most even distribution of light across the retina. The pupil of the eye will get larger or smaller according to the intensity of the light. Sight, therefore, should be considered an "alerting" process, one that triggers the eye to prepare itself for the process of vision.

2. **Acuity** is the result of all the actions that have to take place in the eye to provide for clarity of the image that the light presents on the retina. The two eyes align, and the focusing system of the lens adjusts to bring the light onto the retina. Acuity, therefore, is a "sorting" or "adjusting" process that allows for the best possible signals to be transmitted to the visual centers of the brain via the optic nerve.

3. **Vision** is the total interpretative act for the comprehension of the image as seen by you. Vision is dependent not only upon the image that has been clearly seen but also upon your history—by the context into which you place the image. Vision, therefore, is the learned interpretation of the visual signals that have been presented to the brain. It is more dependent upon your particular experience than it is on the actual physical structure of your eye, although the physical health of the eye can certainly enhance or delay vision.

When you are asked to read an eye chart to see if you have 20/20 vision, what is the doctor really testing?

You have probably been asked to to sit in a chair and look all the way across the room at an eye chart on the wall. The chart usually has letters on it that are larger on the top of the chart—it always begins with that gigantic letter *E*—and get smaller as you move, row by row, to the bottom of the chart.

That chart is named for its inventor, a Dutch ophthalmologist named Hermann Snellen, who first began working with his creation in the mid–nineteenth century.

Snellen developed his chart in order to be able to standardize a level of acuity that could be considered the product of an average healthy eye. The first 20 in "20/20 vision" refers to distance; you stand twenty feet from the chart while attempting to read the smallest letters that you can still see clearly. The second 20 refers to the size of the letters. Thus if you are said to have 20/20 vision, you are able to see and comprehend the twenty-point letters at a distance of twenty feet. If you have 20/10 vision, you therefore have sharper-than-usual vision; if you have 20/200 vision, you would be considered nearsighted. That Snellen set the standard distance for his test at twenty feet, the same amount of space that is the adult's usual arena of visual clarity and interest, is certainly no coincidence and attests to the overall excellence of this diagnostic tool.

If you fail to display 20/20 vision, you may be experiencing what an eye doctor would call *refractive problems* with your vision. These include nearsightedness, farsightedness, and astigmatism. (Note that these conditions will be explained in more detail in Chapter 4.) These are conditions for which the conventional doctor will give a prescription for glasses or contact lenses.

Apart from the Snellen chart, there are physical and behavioral indicators if you are having problems with *refraction*, or the way in which your eyes bend light in order to see. Among these are

- Squinting or straining when trying to see objects clearly
- Headaches when you try to read
- Redness or tearing from the eyes after performing a visual task
- Frequently rubbing eyes after performing a visual task
- Feeling fatigued after performing a visual task
- Misinterpreting what you have read or mispronouncing the words you read
- Complaining that you cannot see

All of these issues may relate to refraction. All might require a prescription of glasses or contact lenses in order to balance or correct.

Another primary visual skill has to do with ocular motilities (eye movements). As I said above, there are two basic types of movement: the saccadic, which allows you to move your eyes from one place to another in a scanning motion; and the pursuit, which allows you to target a moving object. Both forms of movement are needed in order for your eyes to move in all three planes of motion, the horizontal, the vertical, and the diagonal.

Examples of the planes of movement include the horizontal motion of the eyes across a line of print in a book and the specific targeting motion that allows your eyes to come to the end of one line of type and move rapidly to the left and down to the beginning of the next line of type. There is also the up-and-down motion that allows you to add up a list of numbers and the near-and-far movements required to copy information from a blackboard at the front of a classroom. Near-and-far movement is also required in sports, as in hitting or catching a ball.

The following are indicators of problems with eye movements:

- Turning your head instead of moving your eyes

- Having a very short attention span
- Continually losing your place on a page of printed material
- Poor orientation skills for placing a drawing on a page
- Omitting words, especially small words, when copying information
- Displaying poor coordination during physical activity

Another vital visual skill is eye teaming, or binocularity. Because your sense of depth in space is largely dependent upon your ability to use your eyes together as a team, if you have issues with eye teaming you are under constant stress to maintain a balance in your nervous system. Tasks that others take for granted, such as driving a car, can be very difficult for you if you have binocularity issues. Signs of poor eye teaming include

- Seeing double images
- Squinting with one eye, closing one eye altogether, or covering one eye with your hand in order to see clearly
- Tilting your head to one side in order to block the vision in one eye or as a student in school, leaning far off to one side of your desk in order to block the vision in one eye
- Blinking excessively
- Having issues with comprehension of what you are seeing, especially if you are performing below your level of skill and intelligence
- Rubbing your eyes very often or experiencing exhaustion after concluding visual tasks
- Reacting inappropriately to objects moving toward you, as in not being able to catch a ball
- Becoming car sick when reading in a moving vehicle
- Needing to hold on to a railing while walking down stairs
- Inability to shop in stores whose aisles are too narrow

Finally, there is the visual skill of focusing, or *accommodation*. This is the ability for your eyes—primarily our lenses—and your brain to be able to sustain attention on one target clearly. It is also a skill of shifting that sustained attention from one target to another while maintaining clarity of image. Without clarity, you cannot identify any target or any object. Without clarity, you cannot separate the target from its background, its environment. Without clarity, you cannot know if an object is moving within its environment, that is, moving toward you or away from you.

Among the signs of issues with accommodation are

- Feeling fatigue when performing visual tasks, especially tasks that require near vision
- Headaches that are located around your eyes
- Seeing print blur as you read
- Seeing letters and lines in books run together or seem to move and jump around

Now, in and of themselves, none of these signs indicates an eye ailment. But all can be important indicators as you seek to balance and improve your vision. In the pages that follow, I will discuss specific vision issues, their underlying meanings, and their cures. But before I can do that, I must first discuss the sense of vision and the eye-brain connection as I have already discussed the physical eye itself.

CHAPTER 2

Vision

Understanding the Image

"You can't behave differently until your eyes perceive things differently."

—Suzanne Dalia

Where sight is a gathering of information at the present moment, vision is a combination of the past, the present, and the future ways we utilize our sight. To borrow from "Star Trek" for a moment, that makes vision something of a space-time continuum.

Where sight is a passive system, the flow of images and light into our brains, vision is dynamic. It is that image put into context, infused with meaning. It is more than observation; it is judgment.

To put it in a simpler way, vision is our ability to take meaning from our environment. It is pervasive in everything we see, touch, and do. It is a reflection of our biases, our hopes, and our judgments, all in one package.

Because vision is dynamic, it involves change. We change by viewing new things and by putting those new images into the context of what we have viewed previously.

More, vision involves a dynamic relationship between the being that sees and the being that is seen. That which we view changes by having been seen. Modern physics has proven that even the smallest particles of matter actually change their patterns of behavior when they are being observed. The act of being observed elicits a change in all things. Thus, everything shifts by the act of seeing.

Vision as an energetic system varies depending upon what is seen. If we look at a chair, does that chair actually change its structure, its self, when we are looking at it? No, at least not in any way that can be specifically measured. But if we look at a person, animal, or any other living thing, depending upon the energy we bring into our gaze, we can have a profound impact upon that living creature by just seeing it.

Scientific evidence would have us all believe that we can impact each other in a positive or negative way through the sense of touch. Studies have shown that touch is a powerful healing tool. There is, for instance, a study of a town in Pennsylvania in which the families had terrible, high-fat diets, eating the worst possible foods every day. But what made this town unique was that they were so healthy in spite of their diets. And what the study showed was that many of the people in this community were related; in fact, they were one big family, and they had formed an extended family with the rest of the community who were not related by blood. These were people who were touching each other, holding each other. And they were healthy people.

Similar studies have shown that the same is true with animals and that our other senses contribute to our well-being as well. The sense of smell, for instance, can be a powerful healing tool, as aromatherapists have shown us.

But we now must place the sense of sight within this category as well. Not only can we improve our vision naturally, but we can also use the sense of sight itself as a healing tool. As our vision shifts, our perception shifts, and with these shifts of perception, our whole life can change. Physical ailments can fall away. Mental and emotional limitations can dissolve. This has certainly proven to be true in the case of newborns who bond with their mothers by deep eye-to-eye contact.

How we are looked at and how we look at others can bring about healing or damage to both parties. How we look at the world—out of angry eyes, loving eyes, biased eyes, judgmental eyes—determines not only who we are but to a large extent, what response we will receive.

It certainly may sound like a tired cliché, but our eyes truly are the windows to our souls. In traditional Chinese medicine, a medical philosophy and practice that has been followed in Asia for more than five thousand years, vision is like breathing; it involves an inward and an outward flow.

The Dynamic Flow

The Inward Flow

Energy and information flow into the eyes from the external world, but some people do not like the images that they are receiving and thus limit their perception of their external environment. In other words, people do actually see exactly what they want to see—nothing more, nothing less. There are those who travel through the world wearing blinders. In fact, those who habitually choose not to see the world around them may gradually reduce their field of vision by developing physical conditions, like glaucoma, that will allow them not to see.

Others choose to blur their personal image of the world, so that they can avoid seeing the tiresome details of life while still being able to see the grand picture, albeit in a somewhat smudged manner. They tend to enjoy living in a pleasant haze, avoiding dealing with or looking at the total truth of life but never fully withdrawing from it. This adaptation can lead to physical conditions like cataracts, which create a dulling of vision.

Those who concern themselves too much with details may alter the image of the external world they are receiving. They restrict their concentration to the area immediately surrounding themselves, which adaptation may lead to either nearsightedness or lack of depth perception.

The Outward Flow

We can often recognize people's emotional state simply by looking into their eyes. The emotions recorded there—love, hate, anger, grief, and worry among them—not only reside there but push forward from those eyes into the world. It is as if there were an outward stream of energy and solid information shooting forth, traveling into the eyes of others around them. Some people seem to consciously make use of the exchange of energy between persons in order to manipulate others. Some try to use eye contact to dominate others. Still others try to dump their negative emotions, their fear, aggression, and bitterness, onto others. Some use eye contact as a means to drain others of their energy.

If indeed this outward flow of energy exists, it may be that those who use it to express bitterness or anger or to dominate others create a pressure in their eyes. This pressure may, in time, translate into inflammations, such as conjunctivitis, or into raised intraocular pressure, as in glaucoma. However, if the outflow through the eyes is blocked or suppressed, the pressure building in the eyes will be expressed through tears, either through the almost total suppression of necessary tears, resulting in dry eyes, or through eyes that water nearly all the time.

Thus, in order to be healthy, we humans need both aspects of the flow of vision to fully and appropriately connect us with our world and those in it. Our vision must be like our breathing, in and out.

But what remains is to identify the aspect of ourselves that is behind the dynamic flow known as vision. And that aspect, that organ, is not the eye. The simple truth is that the eyes themselves transmit, but they do not see. Only the brain truly sees. Just as the video camera that recorded your last trip to Paris could not have possibly known to record the Eiffel Tower, your eyes need your brain to enact the role of tourist-at-large in the world in order to be directed as to just what to look at and transmit. The recording part is happening inside the brain, too. Because at its most effective, vision involves more than transmitting an image. It involves cognition.

Vision and Cognition

Just as there are specific skills required in order for the human eye to see, the act of *cognition*, or understanding, demands three specific skills on the part of the brain so that the image seen translates into the image understood.

These brain functions, called *cognitive skills*, are

- The ability to identify the visual stimuli
- The ability to discriminate the visual stimuli
- The ability to integrate the visual stimuli

These functions are perhaps best understood when compared with the machine that mimics the human mind—the personal computer. Think of this eye-brain connection rather like the virus program that you have on your computer. You load information from a floppy disk, but before it is added to your hard drive and put to use, it is scanned and checked to be sure that the information contained on the disk is of a type that is comprehensible to your computer's operating system and that it presents no sort of threat. In the same way, when the image input by your eyes travels to your brain, it must first be checked before it can be put to use. First, the image must be identified and placed into some kind of context. Second, it must be judged; the brain must be sure that this is an image that should be stored for present and future use—in other words, added to the overall pool of images as part of a future context for other things seen and judged. Finally, if the image is selected, it is absorbed, or added to that pool of knowledge, that personal hard drive in your brain.

To be sure, not all images pass through all three levels of cognition. Many images cause the brain to ask, "What is that?" This may occur if the image is not received correctly by the brain, it is blurred, or if in any other way it does not come through the eyes efficiently. Or the image may be clear and precise as it passes through the eyes, but the brain does not have the ability to correctly process what it has seen. If either part of the vital eye-brain mix breaks down, the process of comprehension dissolves.

Research: The Eye-Brain Connection

Research studies on patients born with congenital cataracts have been of vital help in our understanding of the complexities of the eye-brain connection. The cataracts caused these patients to be blind from birth. After they grew to young adulthood in a blind state, they at last underwent an operation that removed the cataracts and allowed them to see. After the operation the patients' visual acuity was very good; that is, their eyes were able to receive and transmit images clearly. But they were not able to identify anything that they were seeing. They were often not able to make such simple identifications as the difference between a square and a circle. However, if they were allowed to trace the outline of a shape with their fingertip, they were immediately able to identify its shape. It often took hours for these patients to learn the ability to sort, judge, and absorb new information. And researchers found that the older the patients at the time of the operation, the harder it was for them to learn. Most never achieved the skills necessary to read.

One such case of a patient with congenital cataracts is recorded in Arthur Zajonc's book *Catching the Light: The Entwined History of Light and Mind*. The patient was an eight-year-old boy who had received an operation to cure his blindness. About him, Zajonc writes

> Following the operation, they were anxious to discover how well the child could see. When the boy's eyes were healed, they removed the bandages. Waving a hand in front of the child's physically perfect eyes, they asked him what he saw. He replied weakly, "I don't know." "Don't you see it moving?" they asked. "I don't know," was his only reply. The boy's eyes were clearly not following the slowly moving hand. What he saw was only a varying

brightness in front of him. He was then allowed to touch the hand as it began to move; he cried out in a voice of triumph, "It's moving!" He could feel it move, and even, as he said, "hear it move," but he still needed effort to see it move. Light and eyes were not enough to grant him sight. The light of day beckoned, but no light of mind replied within the boy's anxious, open eyes. The light of nature and of mind entwine within the eye and call forth vision.

Since the 1950s, other studies have shown the effect of visual deprivation on the eye. From birth, some monkeys were raised under conditions of extreme visual deprivation and were in total darkness for the first eighteen months of life.

When these poor animals were finally brought out into the light of day, they exhibited complete functional blindness. They stumbled, they fell, they seemed totally incapable of performing the most basic visually directed behaviors.

When the animals' eyes were tested, they were proved to be not functionally but structurally blind. The total lack of light stimulation during the important development period of their first eighteen months of life had resulted in degeneration of their eyes to the point of total blindness. The test proved that light stimulation in the environment is essential to the development of normal visual perceptual abilities.

Another experiment with monkeys allowed the animals a few hours a day of diffuse light stimulation. But other than those few hours, the monkeys were again raised in total darkness for the first eighteen months of life.

At the end of this study, the monkeys proved to be functionally blind. But they were not structurally blind; their eyes had not deteriorated to the point of blindness. The diffuse light had allowed the animals' eyes to develop physically, but the animals had not developed a context to allow them to understand or make use of what they were seeing.

These studies, although grotesque in nature, are vital to our understanding of human development. They prove that the early experiences of children shape the functional organization of their brains and determine how well they will be able to process and make use of information as they grow to adulthood.

We have now learned a bit about how the eyes and brain work together during the vital developmental stages of childhood. But how can these cognitive skills be relearned in adults who have lost their inborn skills due to catastrophic illness, and how may we help those who have never learned to work to their fullest capacity? Some insight into this conundrum may be found in the following study.

Like many a brilliant scientist, G. M. Stratton, the author of this study, was also a bit of a madman. In the late 1800s, he set forth to explore his own powers of adaptability and cognition. To do this, Stratton outfitted himself with a highly unusual pair of glasses. These glasses contained a prism to bend the light as it entered his eyes so that the image that he saw with both his eyes was upside down. Not only was it upside down, but it was also backward. And Stratton wore these glasses for several weeks for all his waking hours.

At first he found that simple tasks, such as walking down steps or picking up a glass, were all but impossible. He also found himself in a constant state of nausea and confusion.

After a few days, Stratton's nausea began to wane, his confusion to lift. He found that his mind began to adapt to his new environment as perceived through his glasses. Over time, Stratton was able to perform the simple tasks that had eluded him early on. He was able to walk unassisted if he was very careful. He was able to locate and lift objects from a tabletop. And, as more time passed, he began to actually feel comfortable within his new environment.

Stratton is often misquoted as having said that over time the world seemed to turn right side up and frontward again, but this was not his real conclusion. He said that he always perceived some sense of inversion, no matter how long he wore his special glasses but that he found that his personal visual perceptual system—his own mind— was capable of adapting to that wildly reorganized stimulus input. In fact, Stratton concluded, his mind was at last able to reorganize itself to deal with his new environment as if it were normal.

We may conclude from this research that if the eye is given the opportunity to develop correctly and if the eye-brain connection is properly developed in a child's early years, then the two, working together, have a nearly infinite ability to adapt and grow—to learn.

In fact, we may conclude that all vision is learned. We have to learn to focus our eyes on a target, we have to learn to converge our eyes to work together, and we must learn that the image placed on our retina needs to get attention from our brain in order to have meaning. As an ancient Arabian ophthalmologist put it hundreds of years ago, "The eye cannot see what the mind does not know."

Vision in Traditional Chinese Medicine

To the practitioner of traditional Chinese medicine, the human body is an organic unit with tissues and organs that are both interrelated and mutually dependent. The eyes, being the optical organs of the human body, are both influenced by and influence each and every other organ in the body. Traditional Chinese medicine extends the idea of vision beyond the simple eye-brain connection to an eye-body connection.

More than five thousand years ago, Chinese philosophers and practitioners developed what is called the *wu hsing*, or the five element sys-

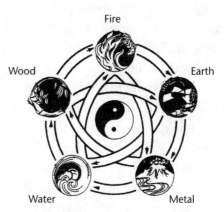

Reprinted with permission from *Feminine Healing* by Jason Elias and Katherine Ketcham. New York: Warner Books, 1995.

tem in order to illustrate and understand the full functioning of the
human system. Within this system, all the parts of the human system
relate to a basic element of nature. And each of these elements—
wood, water, fire, earth, and metal—depends upon the others. All life,
in fact, human and otherwise, depends upon a delicate balance and
interdependence.

In traditional Chinese medicine, emphasis is placed on patterns
in body and mind functions, just as Western medicine places its emphasis on physical structure. Thus, where Western medicine tends to
define illness in terms of functional and pathological processes, the
Chinese believe that both physical and emotional dysfunctions are
due to an imbalance of energies that flow throughout the system con-
necting these interrelated organs.

Considering vision from the standpoint of the five elements and
traditional Chinese medicine, we see that all conditions that inhibit the
correct flow of vision between the eye, the brain, and the being are
either an excess or deficiency in energy as it relates to each of the specific elements.

In my own practice, I find that an understanding of the five elements allows me a greater understanding of each of my patients and
their own unique needs. Further, it gives me a map to follow in creating a treatment protocol for that patient, one that is truly "wholis-
tic" in that it brings into equal consideration my patient's physical
being, including his eyesight, as well as his mental, emotional, and spiritual beings, including his sense of vision.

I also think that it is important for my patients to understand the
philosophy of the five elements. As they find themselves resonating
with one type more than the others, they often can come into an understanding of their own strengths and weaknesses, their own core motivations. This understanding can empower sufferers with an ability to
change past patterns and to free themselves from negative motivations.

Take a look at each of the following five elements and the human
type that each illustrates. See if you can find yourself anywhere among
the five.

The Wood Element

The liver and the gallbladder are the human organs that are most often associated with wood, with the liver being the organ that is most closely related to the eyes. Your liver determines how well your eyes function. The liver controls the state of the tendons that directly impacts the capacity for contraction and relaxation, which is important to vision. The liver is also responsible for regulating and dispersing the flow of life energy (called *qi*, or *chi*) throughout the whole body and the eyes.

The *hun*, or soul, is related to the wood element and to the liver. It is associated in Chinese texts with intuition, imagination, and the processes of the right side of the brain, just as the element earth is related to the left side of the brain and its analytical functions.

The wood element is linked to the ability to plan and to make decisions. This element also relates to the main themes that play out in our lives. It enhances the ability to see the overall pattern of existence. Therefore, when the wood energy is out of balance, a patient becomes frustrated and angry—the two emotions most associated with the wood element and with the liver.

Many persons who are the wood type feel an inner restlessness. They feel filled with pressure that needs release. They tend to achieve release of this pent-up energy through sudden, unplanned actions. They tend to live and work at high speed. They tend to be impatient because everything else in their environment seems to be moving so slowly.

If wood types give in to this need for speed and action, they will tend to make poor decisions in life, decisions that are not so much based on their actual needs but instead based on their perceived need for a fast decision.

When wood energy is blocked and wood types cannot "see" the path for their life, they quickly begin to feel a lack of direction, creativity, and self-expression. This leads to feelings of depression and frustration. Wood types are sensitive to feeling blocked or obstructed, although it may be said that they often create these situations for themselves. Those who are deficient in wood energy may display physical symptoms as well, including allergies, insomnia, and chronic neck and shoulder pain.

When a patient displays an excess of wood energy, on the other hand, they tend to become "overly yang," which is to say they act rashly, become overly aggressive, tend to behave as the proverbial bull in the china shop. They may exhibit physical ailments as well, from migraine headaches to digestive disorders to cramped muscles.

Wood energy is naturally expansive. It is future-oriented. It is the element of growth, birth, and self-expression. Wood types like to move, to travel, to change. In addition, they may be very impatient with themselves and their need for personal growth and development. But as the wood types truly develop and grow, they see the need for balance in their lives, specifically the need for balance between freedom and responsibility.

In terms of physical vision issues, the wood element corresponds to the ability to visualize. Stagnated wood energy often expresses itself in nearsightedness. When the wood energy moves out of balance, the resulting condition is often one of convergence excess, when the two eyes tend to turn inward, resulting in systemic stress.

The Water Element

Remember that in Chinese medicine all organs are interrelated; they influence and are influenced by one another. The kidneys are said to receive and store all the essences of all the other organs. *Essence* means the original material, that which forms the basis of the tissues, what in Western medicine would be called DNA.

The kidneys are associated with the flow of all fluids in the body. In the eyes, they relate to tears and the aqueous humor that largely makes up the eyes.

The water element relates also to the bladder, which itself represents the storage and conservation of energy, making energy available to the whole system when needed. If the stored energy gets depleted, then the whole being may be exhausted, as it contains no reserves of strength.

The water element relates to will. Will is the ability to focus attention and energy on a specific goal, with the concentration and determination to achieve that goal. If a person is deficient in water energy, the whole being will have difficulty in either starting or completing tasks. That person will be easily discouraged emotionally as well. Those deficient in water energy may also become discouraged with themselves in their feelings of weakness and failure. They may display such physical symptoms as loss of appetite, prematurely wrinkled skin, and brittle joints and bones.

If the water energy is high, a sensation of dryness may extend throughout the being. These people will have a dry nose and throat and will lack perspiration. They may have other physical symptoms as well, including bladder and kidney problems and chronic pain in the lower back.

On the other hand, if water types properly maintain their stored energy, they will be tireless workers. They have the ability to fully achieve their goals.

Water as an element relates to fear. Fear is at the root of many of the type's life troubles: fear of failure, fear of loss of control, fear of responsibility, fear of being dependent, fear of being alone, fear of death, and so forth.

In terms of vision, water types will often have troubles with accommodation (focusing on a specific visual object). They will have trouble trying to identify what is right in front of them.

The Fire Element

The element fire in Chinese medicine is associated with the heart and small intestine. It is also related to what in traditional Chinese medicine is called the *pericardium/triple heater*, what Western medicine calls the endocrine system. This system of glands is responsible for heating and cooling the entire system. Altogether, the organs associated with fire bring blood to the whole body, including the eyes.

Fire represents spirit. It brings energy to the physical body, to the emotions, and to the energy system that runs throughout the human system. It is also said to feed the mind. This spirit includes all the conscious awareness that occurs within the human system and in the world around us. This spirit, therefore, connects each of us to one another and to our whole earthly environment. The stronger the spirit within an individual, the stronger that person's sense of oneness with all creation and the greater the feeling of joy, love, and total bliss.

The emotion associated with the element fire is love. When fire is low, it is hard for fire types to feel loving, since love for them equates with vulnerability. In times of low energy, this vulnerability is to be avoided and the awareness of the spiritual connection with creation breaks down, leaving fire types with a deep sensation of emptiness.

The fire energy is expansive in nature; in itself it knows no limits or boundaries. It has a deep need to express itself through direct communication with others by sharing ideas and feelings. Ask these people about their lives or their work, and you will immediately feel their strong personal energy and the excitement with which they fill their lives.

The people with an excess in fire often find themselves having difficulty in concentrating and paying attention. With a natural intuitive, creative, and even artistic nature, they tend to move through life without a plan. Often they feel that the circumstances of their lives are out of their control. They tend to both feel and behave in an unstable manner. Persons of this type are often given to intense mood swings and bouts of free-floating anxiety.

Along with this emotional instability, people of this type often display a physical instability as well. They tend to be awkward in their movements, clumsy, and they tend to accidentally drop and break things.

Because of their emotional and physical difficulties, which may often be summed in an ongoing desire to move, children of this type are often diagnosed with attention deficit disorder (ADD). Learning skills are further hampered in this type by the wide range of vision issues that they commonly experience. Visually, nothing is easy for them.

Just as in both their bodies and minds, the issues concerning the eyes of the fire type also relate to movement—in this case, to eye movement skills. Those of this type may combine issues with poor focusing skills, poor eye teaming, and poor movement skills. They also lack the ability to make eye contact with others. It can therefore be concluded that those with issues of the fire element have trouble with visual communication, being unable to understand what is seen and to express what has been understood.

The Earth Element

The element earth is associated with the spleen and stomach. This element is responsible for nourishing the eyes.

Earth represents mother—not only physically, by its ability to nourish the body, but also emotionally, by providing both physical and emotional security. The capacity for caring and for providing a stable home for loved ones is especially strong in earth types. They are solid, warm, and pleasant, unless the earth energy is blocked within, causing them to feel empty, unable to nourish themselves or others.

This is the element of the rational mind, the analytical part of the self, the left brain and its processes. The earth element deals with day-to-day matters. It is the thinking part of each individual. When this element gets out of balance, when individuals have too much earth energy, they tend to overthink, to become crippled in their own mind. It can lead to the sensation of an ongoing internal chatter. It can, in extreme cases, lead to obsessive-compulsive disorder.

If one were to ask earth types to describe themselves, they would say that they are sympathetic and caring. And indeed they are. Earth types are among the most supportive people. They universally have trouble shaping the word "no" with their lips. They tend to be very patient with others and willing to listen to other people's heartaches. They also consider themselves to be wonderful friends, loving parents, and, in general, spokespersons for peace, harmony, and cooperation for all the peoples of the world. But it is their very virtues that create their health issues. In their eyes, no matter their color, no matter the gender or age of the earth type, you will see a look of deep concern that has come upon them from their ongoing mission of providing nourishment to all those who hunger. For, what earth types tend not to say about themselves, or even not to know about themselves, is that underneath all the harmony and cooperation is a good deal of insecurity and, often, a great deal of anxiety as well.

The earth types' desire for harmony can be easily thrown off balance when harmony is lacking in the environment. And they tend to have a real knack for getting involved in situations in which all positive emotions are lacking. These situations—family fights, especially—drain earth types of their natural nourishing energy. The more the situation at hand is out of harmony, the more earth types will seek to use their own energy to heal the situation, and the less they will use that energy for their own nourishment. Left unchecked, this pattern leads to disharmony and illness. Among the many conditions common to this type are weight gain; water retention, especially in the abdomen, hips, legs, and ankles; headaches, accompanied by a sensation of heaviness and aching eyes; fibroid tumors; and bowel disorders, including diarrhea, constipation, and distended abdomen.

Emotionally, earth types tend to suffer from worry. It is their core emotion, the sensation that something bad is about to happen. Most often the emotion will manifest itself concerning a loved one and not the earth type himself.

In terms of vision, when earth is out of balance, both the lens of the eye controlling focusing and the ocular muscles controlling convergence become stressed, leading to eyestrain and an ongoing sense of fatigue. It may also result in nearsightedness.

The Metal Element

Metal relates to the lungs and large intestine, the organs that control our ability to let things go and when we will let them go.

In Chinese philosophy, the *po*, which is said to be the corporeal soul, is linked to the element metal. The corporeal soul is the densest and most physical aspect of spirit, as it resides in the physical body. It is said to be the foundation on which the physical body exists and by which it heals. It is what metaphysicians call the etheric body.

This is the element that is responsible for breath, the energy of flow, which connects the individual to the energy outside her body. Each breath connects people inside themselves with the world outside. Because of the rhythm of breath, no human can disconnect from the world, no one can shut off or withdraw from life.

Metal is the element responsible for the formation and dissolution of emotional attachments as well. These bonds between people are the energy that connects each person to the object of attachment. For example, the energy may connect a child with his teddy bear, a husband to his wife. Thus, the core issue for the metal type is relationships, his relation to others, to self, and to the universe.

Relationships can be very difficult for the metal type to successfully enjoy. This is often due to the type's natural tendency to be somewhat rigid in both thinking and personality and because the metal type tends to be a natural critic. Look for metal types to enter a room and immediately inform you that the painting over the mantle is crooked and that the room itself is too warm. Those who share their lives with metal types often feel as if they were being constantly criticized and controlled.

Yet what others do not see is that people of the metal type tend to demand even more from themselves than they do from others. They tend to hold themselves up to impossible standards and to take upon themselves not only their own well-being and that of their family, but of the whole world as well.

Metal types are natural workers. They tend to be drawn to jobs of great responsibility and to give those jobs their all. Their weakness in work is that they often become so absorbed in the organizational details that they lose sight of core issues. They can ultimately forget why something was so important to them and cling only to the fact that it seems important. As they become more and more rigid in their thinking, they become increasingly vulnerable to anything that may be considered spontaneous. Anything that does not fall into their personal pattern of order can become confusing, frustrating, and, ultimately, frightening.

Obviously, metal types like to be in control. They have the tendency to be overbearing. They are judgmental and critical of others. In short, they are addicted to being right. Their greatest fear is losing control. Second to this, their other great fear is that their mission in life of bringing order to global chaos will somehow be corrupted.

Rigidity is the key to many of the physical ailments of the type. They often experience chronically stiff and tight muscles and have a marked inflexibility of the spine, especially of the neck. Breathing problems are also common, from chronic sinus infections to asthma. Metals are given to allergies as well, especially to animal dander and chemicals in the environment.

In terms of vision, metal types again are all about relationships. Proper vision relates to an understanding of where things are in space and to spatial organization of the things that are part of the environment. It also relates to eye teaming and binocularity. When the metal element is out of balance, there is a sense of chaos in an individual's world, in both their physical environment and their internal emotional landscape. Metal types commonly lose the ability to find themselves in the universe and to have the universe wrap itself around them in a manner that makes sense. They also tend to have poor eye teaming and poor binocularity.

An Exercise in Balance

Balance may certainly be said to be the key for the elements. Each of us balances all five elements within our being. But each of us, as well, more strongly resonates with one element than with the other four.

And in this way, the five elements give us a map to follow. If we can identify ourselves among the five types, we will have a knowledge of our own strengths and weaknesses that can guide us through life.

I am often asked if it is possible to be more than one type. And, in my practice I have often seen that it is quite possible for a patient to combine the traits of two separate types. Combination types should learn to understand both patterns in terms of their own lives and try to come to understand both how those patterns were put in place and under what circumstances each pattern takes dominance over the other. In this way, even the complexities of the combination type can be helpful as guideposts on the path to healing.

In my office, I have often found the five elements to be a powerful tool for diagnosis and treatment, as illustrated in the following case study.

Patricia, the Nurse Who Could Not Trust

When I first met Patricia she was a forty-eight-year-old married woman with more than twenty years' professional nursing experience. Her husband was a teacher in the local school system. I knew them both because her husband had, over the years, referred many of the children that he taught to my practice—children who displayed varying degrees of learning difficulties. After he saw the results of the work I had done with the children, he referred his own wife to me. Before her first visit, he told me that she had always been a slow reader, and that reading made her very sleepy.

I examined her eyes and found them both to be very healthy. She required no prescription for distance vision and only a moderate lens for near. Her chief complaint to me was that her eyes got very tired whenever she read and that she had bags under her eyes.

While I didn't think that there was much I could do for her cosmetically, I explored with her the nature of her issues with reading. She told me that often, when she read, the print on the page would go in and out of focus, and that she often had to read and reread the material. She seldom could understand what she read on the first try. She said that she had liked to read as a child, but the trouble began in her later years in school. By the time she was in college, she was able to take only one or two courses a semester because the reading required by more classes would overwhelm her. During that time, she became aware of how poorly she learned from the printed page and how much more effectively she learned from lecture presentations. She began to tape her lectures and listen to them as a way of learning that circumvented the printed page.

My examination of Patricia, however, revealed more than just a reading problem.

In evaluating all the components of vision, I found that she had issues both with her focusing and her eye-teaming skills. I explained to her that difficulties like these had more far-reaching results than just problems with reading and that they affected her ability to know what she was looking at and where objects were in relation to her.

Patricia did not know how to orient herself in the world. And with these parts of herself out of balance, she was not able to effectively communicate what she was experiencing and feeling. She had already told me that she had problems giving or taking directions when it came to locating a place in space. She also could not read a map. This was due to the fact that she could not visualize a locale in space. As we talked more, she revealed more and more issues that she had not only with vision but with spatial relationships as well. For instance, she revealed that she wore her wristwatch on her right wrist, not because she was left-handed, but because she could never remember her left from her right.

Where other eye examinations might have simply shown Patricia's eyes to be perfectly healthy and given her a stronger prescription for near vision, mine had revealed her difficulty with eye teaming, an issue that had limited her for years. And further, it gave her a solution, a plan of action.

I explained to Patricia that eye teaming can be a learned skill if it does not come naturally. Even in middle age, it was not too late to develop an increased quality of vision.

But before we put together a plan for Patricia, I felt that it was important to go deeper with her case and to discuss the emotions that underlie her vision difficulties.

I told her that seeing the world the way she did made it difficult for her to trust either herself or the world around her. It had led to feelings of suspicion and the ongoing need to verify the things in her life. Often, Patricia had adapted to learn to trust things by the sense of touch or by talking to herself, convincing herself that she had identified correctly. Sometimes she would look at things again and again, in order to be sure of what she had seen.

Patricia agreed with all that I had said and volunteered that this lack of trust extended to her emotions as well. She had always had issues with trusting her husband, although he had never given her any reason for suspicion and had even turned to therapy to resolve her trust issues.

We began our work.

The first step was to have Patricia come to realize that far from not working hard enough or pushing herself enough, a great deal of her issues with vision had to do with pushing too hard and working herself to exhaustion. I felt that it was important Patricia begin her vision work with an atmosphere of experimentation and informal fun. If Patricia could judge herself and her efforts less and simply experience what was right before her eyes more, she could accomplish a great many of her goals with less effort and more enjoyment of life.

I put together for Patricia a home-based program of exercises. For a total of nine months, she worked hard, mixing and matching a series of exercises based not only on Patricia's vision issues, but on her character as well. Some exercises were done every day, some every other day, some only weekly. Through the whole process Patricia and I stayed in close touch.

At the end of nine months, Patricia was able to read much more easily and to retain what she had read. Perhaps equally important to her, the bags under her eyes had disappeared as she stopped pushing herself so hard.

Midway through her work, she began playing tennis, at first as a part of her vision therapy and then later for fun and exercise. She found that as weeks passed, she was able to see and return the ball much more easily, so that the activity had actually become fun.

At home, she reported, she found that she felt more relaxed and centered. Because she had reached the point at which she felt safe in the world and felt that she could trust her environment, she had also learned to trust herself. In doing so, she also began to trust her beloved husband, which led to a renewal of their relationship.

Mental Symptoms and Vision Conditions

As you saw in the case above, Patricia's problems could not be contained in a single box. Because she had trouble seeing, she had trouble understanding. And because she had to struggle every day to see and understand, she had also developed the emotional issue of lack of trust.

What affects one part of us ultimately affects the whole. Virtually all vision issues have ramifications in our minds and hearts, and this has led vision professionals to the development of behavioral optometry and vision therapy, a field of study that has been around for only about sixty years.

This expanded area of the practice of optometry looks at vision from a holistic point of view, working toward changes in awareness and not just sight, with the alteration of both perception and behavior in order to achieve lasting vision improvement. Behavioral optometry works from the idea that the symptoms that vision disorder sufferers commonly report—headaches, blurred vision, tired and itchy eyes, and the like—have more than a hereditary or pathological cause. These problems can be due to various physical, psychological, postural, and/or lifestyle stresses that are part of an individual's everyday life. These can be changed through proper training and increased awareness.

Like traditional Chinese medicine in the East and homeopathy in the West, behavioral optometry sees each patient as an individual who manifests the ailments as a whole being. Therefore all the symptoms of that individual are a part of that whole. The imbalances of that individual's life are to be supported and addressed, rather than distorted and suppressed. For this reason, behavioral optometrists are far less likely to give prescription lenses—the all-purpose drug of the average optometrist. And when they do give prescription lenses, behavioral optometrists tend to give them in far lower potencies than do their counterparts in optometry.

Beyond this, the behavioral optometrist believes that there are many disorders that respond well to this form of vision treatment that would not respond at all to standard optometrics. Some of these ailments include reading and learning problems, especially early learning issues; attention deficit disorder, attention deficit–hyperactivity disorder, and a host of other behavioral problems; burning, itching eyes; eyestrain or visual fatigue; traumatic brain injury; stroke and its aftermath; chronic fatigue; faulty convergence and focusing problems; and the often overlooked issues with eye teaming and vision suppression.

As people begin to change behavior patterns, specifically those linked with vision, they discover that their visual behavior is directly linked to their general behavior and that the whole system must be rebalanced in order to effect the appropriate visual changes. In other words, the subtle focusing miscue may have major ramifications on the level of personality and perception. As the visual pattern changes, so will behavioral patterns. And as general patterns of life shift, so will vision patterns. The whole system will always seek balance, not only for itself but for all of its parts.

This process reinforces the use of the word *therapy* in vision therapy. Psychology has been part of optometry for many years now, through the fact that vision is physically connected to the human organs of perception. Thus vision is an aspect of human perceptual phenomena. And thus the two fields of psychology and optometrics naturally overlap. The specific field of behavioral optometry steps even further into the arena of psychological study by moving beyond the mere mechanics of the eye to stress the process of vision.

It has been noted again and again that the actual physiological optical mechanism of the eye will vary during a problem-solving trial and that people's actual physical requirement for prescription lenses will change during times of stress. Circumstances and emotions can literally shape the physical nature of people's beings, specifically their eyes. Another example of this is the fact, substantiated by research, that those suffering from multiple personality disorder often need different vision prescriptions for different aspects of their split personalities. Is it no wonder that behavioral optometrists insist on taking a holistic viewpoint of their patients?

While in the process of undergoing vision therapy, a person's psychological makeup, that which may be both the cause or the by-product of visual problems, often undergoes tremendous change. But this change is not a one-way street. Vision problems may cause psychological and emotional difficulties, and psychological disturbances may underlie vision issues. In any event, they often mirror each other, one playing yin to the other's yang. Ultimately, as a result of vision therapy, both sets of patterns must break down and change as the person moves toward health.

When asked to define the concept of health, homeopath George Vithoulkas said simply, "Freedom." To me, this is an excellent definition, as it is the job of behavioral optometrists to set their patients free to live their lives to their optimum potential for joy and creativity.

Such was the case with little Michael, a boy who had been labeled as literally "lost in space."

Michael, a Boy out of Balance

Michael was in the fourth grade when he was brought to see me. By that time he had already been complaining for years that he could not see and that his eyes bothered him. He had been taken to doctor after doctor, all of whom said, "He does not need any glasses for seeing. His eyes are completely healthy."

As far as those doctors' statements were concerned, they were correct. His eyes were healthy. Yet, although Michael could see, he could not correctly comprehend what he saw.

At an early age, Michael had also been diagnosed with attention deficit disorder (ADD). This stigma had been placed upon him because of his trouble reading and his short attention span. Although he was nine years old, Michael could not read well. He was good, however, at math and all math problems, except word problems. I had to ask myself, as I always do with those labeled with ADD, does this boy truly have this ailment, or has he been conveniently categorized by the educational system that is seeking a solution for a troubled student?

When I examined Michael's eyes, I found that his brain was not efficiently directing the motion of his eyes. He also showed dysfunction with eye teaming, which applied even more stress to his vision system and made it all the more difficult for him to focus his attention on the teacher at the front of the room.

I also tested Michael's balance and his gross and fine motor skills and found him far behind in development of both. Together, all of these issues wreaked havoc with his ability to pay attention to, absorb, and organize information. On top of this, he was certainly aware of the fact that he was being treated as different, and this treatment was causing him an ongoing sense of anxiety that he demonstrated with inappropriate behavior in the classroom.

But—and this is important—he did not have ADD. No amount of medication for this condition would do anything more than confuse the case, making it all the worse.

Again, as I do for all my patients, I designed a treatment program specifically for Michael, one that was largely home-based (under the supervision of a parent) but one that also included several office visits, during which Michael was under both my own care and that of a professional vision therapist.

Michael worked hard at his vision therapy for a whole year, during which time his reading and writing skills as well as his overall behavior improved dramatically. He was lucky that he received treatment for his problem at an age early enough that he, unlike Patricia and so many others, would not have to move through a great portion of his adult life without ever achieving what he could.

He was also lucky in not being given the drugs that too many of our children are now being given, in many cases because an underlying vision and perceptual problem is going unidentified. It is important that in the years to come we reclaim the many millions of Michaels, children whose innate gifts go undeveloped because they are shrouded under the amorphous blanket labeled ADD.

In the pages to come, we will explore other cases and ailments as they are considered and treated with vision therapy and behavioral optometry. But first, now that we have discussed the human eye and the mind that both guides and depends upon that eye, let us take a moment to consider what hides behind the mind in the aspect of greater vision: the human soul.

CHAPTER 3

Greater Vision

Beyond the Eye-Brain Connection

"From an eyesight and vision point of view, this dimension of vision,
beyond the sensory state, probably includes the soul."
—Robert-Michael Kaplan,
The Power Behind Your Eyes

When people first come into my office, they quite correctly expect me to check their eyes. Any eye doctor will do that. But there are different ways to check a patient's eyes, different reasons for doing so, and different levels of meaning that I can take from the information within.

In Western medicine it is all pretty cut and dried. A patient goes to a conventional eye doctor with a complaint or a symptom. Something's wrong. The Western physician then searches for the "underlying cause" of that symptom. When he can match the specific symptom and its precise cause, he can very often diagnose a specific disease. Once he has identified the disease, he follows a treatment that is suggested by the diagnosis. In fact, the patient may have several symptoms, and they may extend in their ramifications far beyond the patient's eyes, impacting upon the whole body. But for the sake of the treatment, the physician tends to keep things simple.

Let's take a look at that for a second.

The training of eye care professionals in this country is scientifically comprehensive, and there have been major advances in treatment of eye disease and even in laser surgery to correct nearsightedness, farsightedness, and astigmatism. But the philosophy of treatment is far too narrow. Doctors are still trained to match the individual to the ailment and to follow the prescribed plan of action for that ailment. What eye care professionals aren't learning to do is correct the underlying problem or to treat concomitant symptoms. They are still untrained in ways to strengthen the whole of the patient's being so the patient will not only be free of a particular ailment but will become healthier in general.

Conventional eye care professionals are still treating individual symptoms and hoping for the best. In their training as eye doctors they're taught that once something goes wrong with patients' eyes there is not much that can be done to help reverse the condition. Vision problems are multiplying at epidemic proportions in our society. The eye care industry is a multibillion dollar business. Glasses, contact lenses, and eye surgery are the major tools of that industry. Aldous Huxley wrote in his book *The Art of Seeing*, "if everyone who had deficient vision had broken legs, the streets would be full of cripples."

Patients seek treatment year after year, their eyesight getting worse. Conventional eye care professionals just give them stronger and stronger glasses. Something is wrong with this picture. The same patients go back because their eyes are getting worse; they are seeing less. And yet, those patients reward the doctors with further visits, paying more and more. And what happens? They are prescribed even stronger lenses. Their eyes may actually get worse, and their vision could deteriorate further. What other industry in the world rewards such numbers of people so well for failing so greatly?

Cataracts are present to some degree in nearly all adults over the age of seventy. And these patients are told, "Let's wait until the cataract ripens [gets worse], and then we can remove it surgically." Patients with macular degeneration and glaucoma are told, "We'll watch it and try to keep it under control." The number of children in our schools being labeled learning disabled and/or as having attention deficit disorder (ADD) is increasing every year. Where is the much-needed prevention, education, or rehabilitation? Something is wrong with all of these pictures.

People think that eye problems are just a natural course of life's process, but that is simply not true. Vision can improve. When people are given so-called corrective lenses, they are being sold a false bill of goods. Corrective lenses don't really *correct* anything. Most of the time when people are given glasses, the lenses cause their eyes to become ever more dependent on those lenses instead of their own eyes. Their eyes lose some of their natural flexibility. And further, when people are being sold prescription lenses, they are being sold drugs, usually without their understanding. And yet in truth, lenses put in front of the eyes have as much impact upon the body as do any other form of medication. Eyeglasses impact much more than the eyes. And instead of just giving stronger and stronger prescriptions to combat eye conditions, where is the aggressive prevention program that would allow many eye conditions to be prevented and corrected?

I look at vision the same way that Chinese medicine looks at disease. Eastern philosophy tends to give attention not only to the physiological findings—the symptoms and their cause—but also to a person's psychological patterns in life. All relevant information, including all symptoms and all discernible patterns, are together called the pattern of disharmony.

Chinese medicine does not look for a direct and simple cause and effect in illness. Instead the search is for patterns—lifestyle choices and circumstances that as a whole are moving the patient toward health or illness. The Chinese physician does not ask, "What X is causing Y?" Instead she asks, "What is the relationship between X and Y in this patient's life?"

As with Western modalities like homeopathy, traditional Chinese medicine insists that no single part of a person—that is, no individual symptom of pain or illness—can be understood except in relation to the whole being. Therefore, that symptom is never traced to its cause but is instead looked at as part of a totality, a pattern.

It is this philosophy that I make a part of eye care and is what I think about as I look into a patient's eyes.

Vision and Soul Themes

I believe that the eye is the external representation of the inner soul. Therefore, when your visual patterns are revealed and are placed within the context of your life's patterns of harmony and disharmony, your soul state is revealed.

Most of these themes relate directly to your quality of vision. I believe that if you can come to understand the theme behind the ailments, the places in life in which energy is frozen and where fear has taken hold, then you can do more than have your vision corrected artificially with the use of corrective lenses. You can perhaps make permanent, natural improvement, not only to your vision but also to your whole being.

The most common themes and the path to healing them are listed here:

- A feeling of powerlessness. You need a path toward healing that involves becoming aware of your own personal power. Related conditions include myopia, convergence insufficiency, cataracts.
- A sensation of being trapped, imprisoned. You may also feel confined to a small way of "seeing" on a sense level, as with a condition like cataracts. Your path is to return to the world unfettered, in a state of freedom. Related conditions include myopia, convergence excess, glaucoma.
- Fear of being out of control. Your path is one toward becoming grounded and feeling balanced as the world moves around you. Related conditions include myopia, overconvergence or convergence insufficiency, strabismus.

- Fear of being alone, cut off from other people. The path to health for you involves developing the ability to love others, while maintaining a sense of self and purpose. Related conditions include myopia (especially in its early stages), macular degeneration, cataracts.
- A sensation of being overwhelmed by life, by all that happens. You need a path toward acceptance of circumstances and a sensation of balance through life's intense circumstances. Related conditions include myopia, hyperopia, presbyopia, strabismus, amblyopia, cataracts.
- Fear of the future. You must work with staying grounded in the present. You should work to get in touch with your own innate wisdom. Related conditions include presbyopia, strabismus, amblyopia, cataracts.
- A sensation of accomplishing nothing in life. Your path must lead to a source of physical, emotional, or spiritual nourishment. You must create a new role in life. Related conditions include convergence insufficiency, strabismus, amblyopia.
- An obsession with safety and stability. Your path involves many risks, small ones and large ones. You must let go of fear. Related conditions include myopia, overconvergence.
- Issues with transitions and change. The path is letting go, learning that life is a ceaseless flow. Related conditions include myopia, convergence insufficiency.
- Issues with boundaries. You need understanding of how and when to take on the issues of others in your own life. You need to walk a path of learning what is and is not appropriate in relationships. Related conditions include myopia, convergence insufficiency.
- The need to be in control. This one can be difficult. You must walk a new path, in which you are able to enjoy your organizational skills and ability to make a quick judgment but will not seek to extend these skills into the lives of others. Related conditions include myopia, convergence excess, glaucoma.
- A sensation of being invaded. Boundaries are the issue here as well. You must learn to establish simple boundaries without push-

ing people away. Related conditions include myopia, convergence insufficiency.

This is, of course, a greatly simplified list and one that is far from complete. But the identification of the soul's theme can be used as a powerful healing tool. Suppose you are a water type (see Chapter 2 for introductory information on the five elements) who has issues with nearsightedness and whose soul theme involves the all-too-quick sensation of having your life invaded by others. The following case illustrates just such a person.

Thomas the Loner

Thomas was forty-six years old and had been a science teacher for the past twenty years at the local high school. He was a very creative teacher who always had new and innovative ways of teaching his students. He would get motivated to do projects when it had to do with the classroom, but on his own he didn't get involved with many projects. He seemed to be happy just sitting at home alone and reading as the world went on around him.

A handsome man with sculptured features and deep-set eyes, Thomas was on the thin side, his hair was 70 percent gray, and he had a high forehead.

I noticed also that his clothing had no energy and made no personal statement whatsoever. Most of his clothes were either brown or gray, as if he were trying to be invisible. When I asked, he said he never wore any bright colors.

He didn't exercise much, preferring to watch a good documentary or read a book for relaxation. He had a slight moaning quality to his voice, and when I asked about his physical shape, he complained of a variety of aches and pains: lower back pain, achy knees, feeling cold a lot.

Thomas had lived alone for over twenty years and saw himself as completely self-sufficient, but he was also aware that he tended to emotionally withdraw into a shell at times. Women he had been involved with during various relationships had told him that they never knew what he was ever thinking or feeling, making them feel alone even in the midst of a relationship—not that that was ever Thomas's intention.

He had never been married but had had numerous relationships since he was twenty years old, none lasting longer than a year and a half and most of them less than six months. He didn't mind being alone, but he wanted to be involved in a long-term relationship. He was a pleasant person and had a lot of friends but no really close friends. He felt frustrated with the fact that he had a very hard time getting close to anyone. He said that there was always a point in any of his relationships where his partner wanted to get closer to him and he would either begin to distance himself from the relationship or create a situation in which he would push his partner away. He said that this pattern had been in place since his college years. He had tried psychotherapy at different times for up to a year, but when he got too close to the therapist he would leave. He said he came to see me because he had attended a workshop I led that addressed the relationship of vision to emotional blocks in our lives. He wanted to see if there was anything he could discover about himself through this process.

I asked him if he would be willing to try an experiment. I had him stand up facing me, and I began to walk toward him. I told him to tell me when he started to feel uncomfortable. When I was about three feet away, he said, "That's close enough." I asked him what came up for him as he was being approached. He said that when I was that close he felt like he just wanted to get away. He wanted to run. He felt a visceral reaction that his personal space was being invaded. He said his eyes started to hurt when I got closer, and it was hard for him to breathe.

The eye examination showed nearsightedness, which he had had since he was six years old, and a moderate convergence insufficiency (his eyes' inability to converge at a nearby object) but not nearly bad enough to elicit this type of an emotional reaction.

I explained to him that through a program of greater vision, where we would be able to use his vision as a feedback system to what his soul was scared of, he would learn to at least have the visual ability to let other people get closer to him. I said that as an adjunct to this he should start psychotherapeutic counseling to have a forum where he could express himself. Vision therapy was also important. His sensory system was keeping people away from him unconsciously. So working with his eyes, his mind, his emotions, and his heart at the same time would help him begin to allow people to come closer to him, and his inner self would then be available in relationships.

Thomas began the vision therapy program on a once-a-month basis. He also performed a home-based program of vision exercises on a daily basis. I also asked him to keep a journal, in which he could keep a record of any sort of change in his vision, for better or worse. I told him to call me if he had any problems understanding anything that he was experiencing or if the exercises brought up emotional feelings that he wanted to discuss. I recommended that he join a men's group for emotional support.

Thomas did all that he was asked to do, and more. He worked diligently at his vision therapy and made a conscious effort to notice his old patterns of emotional behavior whenever they reappeared.

His physical visual system developed a good amount of flexibility within three months. Two months after that he began a relationship, and a year and a half later, was married. He now no longer feels that his space is being invaded by those who wish to get close to him.

In our last session together, I repeated the experiment that had begun our therapy. Again I slowly, steadily walked toward him to purposely invade his personal space. This time, Thomas allowed me to walk all the way up to him and place my hand on his shoulder. The anxiety that he felt in that first experiment was no longer there. He felt that he could breathe freely, and his heart was more open.

_____ **A Problem with Sensitivity** _____

Gloria was a forty-year-old visual artist. Thin, with smooth skin and a long, angular face, she was neatly and stylishly dressed and had very finely combed hair.

Married for four years, Gloria and her husband were contemplating having a child, but she felt overwhelmed by responsibility. She said that the world had always seemed to be too big to her, with too much going on and things happening too fast. Too many people were talking at once for her to be able to hear and understand them.

Gloria no longer wanted to leave her house and had most of her clothing and even her food purchases delivered directly to her so that she would not have to go shopping.

By the time Gloria came to see me she was even more sensitive and had developed numerous food allergies and sensitivity to light, temperature, weather changes, and smells. Only the fact that she was financially well off allowed her the freedom to live in her small town and to stay at home and paint.

A friend who accompanied Gloria told me that Gloria's home was like the homes you see pictured in magazines. Everything was perfectly selected and positioned. Everything was perfectly neat and clean. Gloria reported that she kept her house this way because she felt that she needed order in her life. She said that it would bother her terribly if things were not put away correctly.

In fact, Gloria finally admitted that her need for control and order were a large part of the reason that she feared having a child. She had seen in the lives of her friends that children could bring chaos with them, and she knew that her life would never be as simple or as easily contained and controlled again if she had a child. As she was nervous about any sort of situation in which she could not predict or control the outcome, Gloria became more and more anxious as her husband mentioned children. The thought of letting herself enter the unknown world of parenting terrified her.

Gloria's husband was a good-natured carpenter who, to the best of his abilities, tried to understand and cater to her sensitivities. He too was worried about what would happen if they became parents. Yet both of them very much wanted a child.

On her first visit to my office, I examined her eyes and found that she was seeing 20/20 in each eye, both in near and distance reading, but that her sensitivity to the use of prescription lenses was nothing short of amazing. I could not, in fact, complete tests for vision teaming to my own satisfaction because the tests caused her such dizziness and nausea that we both became alarmed. Her symptoms far exceeded any I had previously seen.

I then checked her peripheral vision and found that it was very difficult for her to be aware of motion on her periphery while focused straight ahead of her. It was as if she were wearing a pair of blinders.

When I said this to her, she said that she would like to be able to wear blinders. "That would probably feel very good," she said.

This suggested the path that the vision therapy would take. Gloria would first have to allow herself to be more a part of the world before we could even address the more sensitive issue of eye teaming.

I explained to her that a program of vision therapy would offer her the ability to see more and feel more in the world. Because of her extreme sensitivity, her soul was able to take in only a little of the world at a time, and too much stimuli overwhelmed her nervous system. She compensated for this by creating order around her and controlling her environment.

If she were to do vision therapy, currently suppressed emotions might rise up. It would be important for her to have an active support system as she worked. I also suggested she consider psychotherapy as another source of support. In addition, I recommended that she see a nutritionally oriented physician who could test her for chemical and food sensitivities and who would also put her on a nutritionally sound diet during the period of her therapy.

Finally, I explained the goals of her vision therapy. As I saw it, the core soul issue was one of helplessness. Gloria saw herself as very small in a very large world. Vision therapy was going to offer her the tools she needed in order to better visually integrate with the world around her. As her eyes opened physically, emotionally, mentally, and spiritually, reality would reshape for her so that she would not feel as overwhelmed by the world and exhausted by her need to control it.

Although admitting that she was afraid, Gloria began vision therapy. She said she was frightened of the many changes ahead and of losing control of her perfectly organized life. But her and her husband's desire to have a child proved to be the lure that she needed in order to get the work done.

While I gave Gloria some exercises to do at home, much of her work was done in the office. She came weekly for a period of six months and then twice monthly for another six. Progress was very slow at first. For the first two months, we took very small steps, working only on the simplest exercises, as I found that she would react to some of the exercises in the same manner that she did the prescription lenses in our first visit.

Her whole defense system would rise up against the exercises, as if the simplest routines implied a wholesale change in her life. After our fourth visit, Gloria pulled me aside and said, "I know that you want to help me, but you are giving me too much to do. I'm not ready to get better so fast. Please just give me one exercise a week for home instead of three." So we slowed down. But we kept on working. Gloria impressed me weekly with that fact that no matter how difficult the work, she returned the next week to keep on trying.

By the fourth month, Gloria's field of vision began to open up, and she was more easily able to integrate both physically and emotionally what was going on centrally (directly in front of her) and peripherally (around her). By the sixth month, she felt she was ready to reduce her office visits and also felt that she might be able to consider getting pregnant. During the ninth month of therapy, she took my recommendation to see an acupuncturist and doctor of traditional Chinese medicine who would work with her fertility issues.

At the end of a year of vision therapy, Gloria had improved enough to decrease the frequency of office visits to once a month. She continued her vision exercises daily in her own home.

After another six months, Gloria learned that she was pregnant. Although there were moments of nervousness as the birth of the child neared, Gloria was filled with joy at the birth of her healthy daughter.

Your Eyes and Your Soul's Expression

Eyes often reveal the inner soul through their expression and through the amount of energy that flows from them. When I examine a person, I can see what I call her "pilot light." This sparkle of light in her eyes can range from bright and brilliant to an all-but-exhausted spark—one that tells me that her life force is very low. Consequently, any treatment I give that patient needs to support her vitality as a whole. In homeopathic philosophy, this spark of life force is called *vital force*, which I think is an apt term. Vital force is a measurement for how freely people are moving through their own lives; how much energy they are taking in and how much they are giving out.

A Simple Exercise

When your eyes meet those of another person, from your best friend or partner to a complete stranger, try to see what information you can learn from that person nonverbally, just from his eyes. You can sense the amount of energy pouring from another person's eyes if you consciously allow yourself to. So give it a try. See what you can discover about another person's soul by looking in his eyes. One person may have vacant eyes—eyes that send the message that no one is home. Another person may seem to be shooting rays of energy from his eyes. Another still may seem to be drawing energy into her eyes from yours. Experiment with eye contact and energy exchange. Make sure to notice how you feel as you make these various forms of eye contact and as you directly come into contact with the deepest level of another person's being.

Did you know that your eyes literally light up when you become happy or excited or when you see someone you love? The pupil reflex in your eye literally gets brighter as you give your full attention to something. Conversely, your eyes begin to dull, their light to fade, as the initial excitement fades. If you want to get a sense of someone's inner being through his eyes, gaze softly into and at those eyes. Do not stare or try to penetrate, but simply gaze and allow the person's expression and emotions to flow into your eyes. If you do this you will be able to get a sense of that person's soul.

Eye contact is one of the strongest and most intimate bonds between two people. It involves the communication of emotion on a soul level and can be a very exciting experience. When your eyes meet another person's, an electric charge runs through your bodies. No matter what specific emotions are exchanged, the contact itself creates a basis for an exchange of this energy and the development of a relationship between you.

The exchange of energy between two sets of eyes is very similar to actual physical contact. The quality of the contact is largely determined by the emotional expression of the eyes. Eyes that have a strong, penetrating glance send the message that others should stay away. Eyes with a soft glance invite others to come closer.

This has to do with the difference between *looking* and *seeing*. Looking involves an aggressive and active component that can best be described as "taking in" with the eyes. Eye contact is a function of looking. When you are looking, you actively express your spirit with your eyes. Seeing, on the other hand, is a more passive process, because you allow the visual stimuli to enter the eye and give rise to an image.

Many people avoid using their eyes on the level of looking, just as they avoid eye contact with others. This is a means of self-defense and, often, denial. When a person is using her eyes defensively or self-protectively, she will tend to stare. Staring will cause others to turn away or to avoid eye contact.

Another Basic Exercise

Here is a simple exercise that you can try with a partner. Choose someone for your partner whom you know well and feel that you can trust completely.

Now, sit comfortably opposite each other and using only your eyes and saying nothing, attempt to send a specific emotional message to your partner. Be sure not to use facial expressions or vocal cues. Use only your eyes.

Be sure to take turns sending and receiving messages.
Try to send and receive these messages:

"I love you."
"I hate you."
"Come closer."
"Stay away from me."
"I am looking at you, but my mind is elsewhere."
"You are the most important person in the world."

By doing an exercise like this one with another person, you can
learn to get in touch with those different aspects of yourself that in
the past may have caused you to send mixed messages. In the same
way, you can learn to help draw emotions out in those with whom you
have a real connection. In time, such an exercise can allow you to learn
more about who you are.

Greater Vision:
A Spiritual Philosophy

In his 1974 book, *Rolling Thunder*, Doug Boyd quotes the Native
American medicine man as he speaks of his own life's philosophy in a
manner that is particularly apt for these pages: "The most basic principle of all is that of not harming others, and that includes all people
and all life and all things. . . . Every being has the right to live his own
life in his own way. Every being has an identity and a purpose. To live
up to his purpose, every being has the power of self-control, and that's
where spiritual power begins."

The power of self-control can be thought of as the power to be
able to assume responsibility for ourselves and our actions. At its highest evolution, I believe that it is the power to heal ourselves. There is
an underlying theme common to all forms of ancient and traditional

health: that all human beings have an innate ability to take charge of their own lives and destinies. From that ability to change comes the ability to heal.

In an interview with Bill Moyers in the book *Healing and the Mind*, internist Thomas Delbanco describes an incident that brought home to him this idea of the "whole person" for whom illness can be a meaningful and life-changing experience. When a friend became seriously ill with a strange assortment of symptoms, a much-admired professor agreed to diagnose her problem and suggest a course of treatment.

After her visit with the doctor, we all had our fingers crossed. "Well, what's the prescription?" we asked. She said, "He tells me I've got to get a washing machine. I'm working too hard at home." That was the diagnosis. You don't find the washing machine prescription in many textbooks, but it helped this woman a lot. She was cured, she was brought back to health, she was made whole, if you will, by that prescription.

Similarly, a very intense man came to see me. He had been leading adventure expeditions all over the world and was writing his memoirs. His eyes were bothering him as he wrote. He had already been to many different doctors and had tried a variety of treatments, including glasses, vitamins, herbal medicines, and exercises, but nothing had worked.

I told him to break his workday into segments of no more than forty-five minutes and to take breaks during the day to briefly perform simple vision therapy exercises for eyestrain. I also gave him a pair of reading glasses. But most important, I told him to get a massage before beginning his work each day and to end each day in the hot tub.

And the man got much better.

By going beyond patients' objective symptoms and entering into a discussion with them about their "reason for being," their core identity, their purpose, and their spiritual values, I can give them an opportunity to help themselves. This is the highest purpose of the physician.

Each of us has internal wisdom, what the New Testament calls the "still, small voice." But just trying to get through the day in our modern world is enough for each of us to get out of touch with that voice. Our internal wisdom is mirrored in the world around us, and when we can look beyond ourselves, we will often see ourselves more clearly.

Greater vision gives each of us the opportunity for self-knowledge and self-examination. This, in turn, helps us to shape the valuable skill of self-control. The journey inward gives us the wonderful opportunity to look—really look—to the world around us, not constantly only at ourselves. Then we see the mirror of our internal wisdom all around us, and we feel the creative and loving connection with the world around us.

As the *I Ching* says, "Self-knowledge does not mean preoccupation with one's thoughts; rather, it means concern about the effects one creates."

The person who has achieved a sense of greater vision, therefore, is aware that every action he takes, every thought that he has, every emotion that he feels impacts the world around him. Thus, that person looks outward from within and inward from without, and he sees that the world is never static, never wholly at rest or at peace. The world is always in a state of transformation, as is the self.

As human beings, as beings in transformation, perfect peace and harmony is not possible in every moment of our lives or for extended periods of our life. We must accept this truth and not let the momentary events of the world or our own self-doubt throw us off balance. Then, when we open our eyes, we will see perfect reality. There is no greater vision than this.

CHAPTER 4

Vision and Distortion

Common Vision Impairments

"In order to see, I have to be willing to be seen."
—Hugh Prather,
Notes to Myself

W hen all is working perfectly, as it was meant to, the eye, working in conjunction with the brain and ultimately the soul, gives us a complete picture of reality. But all too often, there is a breakdown in the system and vision does not take place as it should. And with any form of distortion of the image comes a distortion in meaning as well, as reality is reshaped with the image perceived.

The many and various forms of vision impairment can be broken down into two broad categories: *functional* and *pathological*.

Functional ailments are those that occur without any apparent reason. These often chronic conditions cannot be traced to any specific origin—some are apparent from birth and others develop as a person goes through life—or any specific cause. Instead, they simply appear. Some come on suddenly, and others develop slowly over time. Conventional medicine, which is also referred to as *allopathy*, tends to dismiss the cause for these conditions, since it can seem all but impossible to determine, and simply gives the patient a crutch in the form of corrective lenses, and so on, or explains these conditions, including presbyopia, as a part of the normal aging process.

Pathological conditions are those that are part of a specific disease state, such as cataracts, in which part of the lens of the eye becomes opaque. Conventional medicine responds to these conditions as it does any other pathological condition in the body: by identifying the condition through a disease diagnosis and then by following the predetermined course of treatment established for that diagnosis.

In this chapter, I will discuss just what can go wrong with vision, how the image that is received by the brain can be distorted, and what the standard treatment for such a condition will be. In the next chapter, I will go deeper into the issue and discuss the underlying causes for vision impairments—what makes a nearsighted person nearsighted. I will also discuss some alternative options for treatment of common vision conditions.

Functional Conditions

Millions of people worldwide suffer from functional vision impairments. In the United States alone, approximately three-quarters of the population have some form of functional vision impairment. While these conditions are often considered to be less serious than are pathological conditions, since they usually are controlled by the use of prescription lenses, they are common, chronic, and difficult to correct.

Among the most common categories of functional conditions are binocular disorders, eye movement disorders, and refractive problems.

Binocular Disorders (Eye Teaming)

If our two eyes are functioning correctly both individually and as a team, their individual perspectives are blended by the brain into a single image that gives full stereoscopic depth perception. The term *stereo* comes from the Greek word *stereos* which means "firm" or "solid." Stereoscopic depth perception, therefore, refers to a received image in which objects are seen as three-dimensional solids and in which those objects are realistically placed in a three-dimensional world.

It is our sense of depth perception that largely gives us the ability to move about in the world and to survive in it.

Depth perception depends completely upon binocularity, upon how well our two eyes are working together. Although few of us are aware of it, we each have a dominant eye, just as we do a dominant hand (and, likewise, ear and nostril). If one of the two eyes becomes too dominant, if its image overrides that of the other eye in the brain, problems with binocularity develop. In the same way, if an eye "shuts down" and stops receiving all or part of the image, trouble develops.

Less than 5 percent of the total population with vision impairment have issues with binocularity. This group includes those who have lost an eye through physical injury or other cause, those who have the condition known as lazy eye (amblyopia), and those with eyes that turn either inward or outward (strabismus).

To discover how your two eyes perceive the world differently, try this simple exercise:

Experiencing Binocularity

You are going to need a free hand for this exercise, so either hold the book with just one hand or put the book down on the table while you work.

Notice that there is a giant *X* below.

X

1. Sit with this book approximately sixteen inches in front of you, with the *X* in front of your nose.
2. Cover your right eye with your hand. Look at the *X* with your left eye.

3. Now quickly switch your hand to the left eye and notice if the X seems to move to a new position. If so, things are working as they should.

Convergence Excess

Convergence excess is a common functional disorder within the category of binocularity. The conventional definition for the disorder is that the two eyes turn inward toward each other excessively when focusing on an object or looking at details up close.

Those experiencing overconvergence also often experience blurred vision, intermittent double vision, headaches, eyestrain, and fatigue.

Among the many patients that I have treated with this disorder was Jill, a seventeen-year-old high school student who was referred to my office because she was doing well on her school testing but poorly on longer tests, like the SATs. She was also experiencing headaches. Her visual exam showed that she had 20/20 vision in both eyes at distance and near, but when I tested her eye teaming skills, I noticed that she had the distinct tendency to overconverge. I prescribed a pair of reading glasses that would help to take the strain off her eyes while doing close work. I also gave her a series of vision exercises created to help relieve her of stress and to help her eyes become more flexible. After receiving her glasses and beginning her vision therapy, Jill experienced a marked improvement in her standardized test scores.

Convergence Insufficiency

Whenever we have to thread a needle or do any other sort of close or detail work, we call upon our eyes to converge. The muscles tighten and the eyes turn in toward each other, allowing them to maintain their binocularity while targeting an object that is much closer than is usual. Most of us will feel some strain in our eyes when we have to turn and especially hold them inward, but the person with convergence insufficiency finds it very difficult to turn and hold both eyes inward.

Persons with problems with convergence insufficiency tend to also experience blurred or double vision, headaches, eyestrain, burning in the eyes, and excessive tearing.

Scott, a ten-year-old patient of mine, is a perfect example of this type. Although he was a highly verbal child, he did not like to read. He would start out reading and less than five minutes later, his mother would see him get up and start doing something else. After she noticed that she never saw him reading more than a very few minutes at a time, she brought him to me. She reported that she was becoming alarmed because Scott was also having more and more behavior problems at school and had recently failed reading.

I tested Scott's eyes and, like his previous eye doctor, found that he saw 20/20 both near and far. But unlike that previous doctor, I also discovered that Scott had a convergence insufficiency. (Unfortunately, this condition all too often goes unnoticed and untreated by conventional medicine.)

Scott's eyes had great difficulty working together whenever he was called upon to work or read up close. Brief spells of close work caused him intense stress. No wonder he didn't like to read. I explained to Scott's mother that in a case like his, glasses would not be of any help; only through an ongoing program of vision therapy could he overcome this condition.

After six months of vision therapy, Scott's behavior in school had improved impressively, as had his grades. He now had the ability to focus his eyes on a close task for an extended period of time.

Strabismus

Strabismus is the general category for any misalignment of the eyes, regardless of the type of misalignment, its cause, or the age of onset. Both *esotropia*, or "crossed eyes," and *exotropia*, "wandering eyes," are examples of strabismus. It occurs in approximately 2 to 4 percent of the population. The most frequent time of life for strabismus to occur is between one and five years of age, although the greatest number of cases begins when children are between two and three years of age.

Having an eye turn in or out will affect the entire binocular system, and, as such, it impacts upon people's ability to orient themselves in space and in relation to other objects. Many people with strabismus exhibit profound symptoms of disorientation.

Not all the visual fibers in the retina of the eye have to do with seeing. About 20 percent are used to help with balance. We need both the fibers that see and the fibers that help us balance in order to efficiently and accurately relate to the world around us. For people with strabismus, both types of fibers are affected. The condition, therefore, interferes with their ability to see and to balance or orient themselves in the world.

The condition often occurs because something interfered with the people's development in eye teaming. Eye teaming is, after all, a learned skill. When something interferes—anything from a cataract, a head injury, a high fever, or the amount of light stimulation that each eye receives—strabismus occurs. There is often a genetic component to the condition. Since strabismus affects the ability to balance and comprehend, children afflicted with the condition are often slow to reach their development milestones, especially walking and talking.

Esotropia

Technically, *esotropia* is defined as "the inward deviation of the eye;" popularly, it is known as crossed eyes. The condition can be apparent at birth or can be developed at any time during childhood. Esotropia may or may not be directly related to the focusing skills of the eyes, as well as to binocularity.

Accommodative esotropia, or that which impacts upon the focusing mechanism of the eyes, usually develops between ages six months to seven years. It most commonly develops between ages two and three and is most often treated with prescription lenses.

Congenital esotropia, which usually does not affect the focusing of the eyes, is apparent at birth. It is usually corrected surgically.

Although the eye or eyes turn inward, there is no specific nerve or general muscle damage in many cases of esotropia. The imbalance between the eyes is due to a specific faulty muscle.

In most cases of esotropia, the brain—wonderful, complex organ that it is—adapts around the condition so that the person will see as well as possible with the condition. While the eyes tend to turn inward to each other, the brain selects one eye to see straight ahead and the other to do the turning. In this way, the person's vision is as balanced as possible. Therefore, instead of both eyes turning inward some twenty degrees, for example, one eye may actually turn inward forty degrees and the other remain straight.

The same eye may always be the one to turn inward, although in some cases the eyes alternate, with the right eye crossed half the time and the left eye crossed the other half of the time. In cases in which one specific eye always does the turning, amblyopia may develop.

People with esotropia may also experience headaches, eyestrain, problems suppressing the image from one eye, issues with depth perception, and head tilt. Conventional doctors treat esotropia, depending upon its type and severity, with either prescription lenses or surgery.

Exotropia

With exotropia the eyes have an outward deviation (away from each other). The condition can be apparent from birth or can develop at any time in childhood. People experience varying degrees of exotropia, from intermittent, in which the eye turns out only part of the time, to constant and alternating, in which each eye turns out part of the time, to specific. In some cases, the person's eye will turn out only when he is looking into the distance; in other cases, only when he is looking up close. Exotropia may or may not be evident to others, depending upon the degree to which the eye turns and the person's ability to compensate for and adapt to it.

People with exotropia also experience double vision and/or suppression of the image in one eye. Those with intermittent exotropia often develop adaptations that allow them to suppress or ignore the image from the wandering eye and will therefore never experience double vision. During times in which the eyes are focused straight, the suppression will end and both eyes will see normally. If the eye turn is constant, amblyopia, or lazy eye, will likely develop. Light sensitivity is also a common complaint.

As they do with esotropia, conventional doctors turn to prescription lenses or surgery as forms of treatment.

Amblyopia

Amblyopia, popularly called lazy eye, is decreased eyesight that usually affects only one eye. The decreased eyesight is not correctable by prescription glasses. This is not an optical problem; there is nothing physically wrong with the eye to cause the weak vision. The problem occurs when the brain ignores some of the information that is being input by the eyes.

It is believed that amblyopia develops in the visual pathway between the eye and the brain and is due to disuse of the eye during the all-important period of development between birth and age seven. It can most often occur when there is a constant turn of an eye or if there is a great deal of difference between the prescriptions required by each eye. It is important to note that amblyopia has nothing to do with an eye turn or a wandering eye, but a lazy eye may result in people whose eyes do turn or wander. If a person's eye turns in or out, his brain may selectively choose to ignore the image from that eye, in order to avoid double vision. In time, the person's nervous system may habitually ignore the image of that eye if the eye turn remains in place after the person is eight or nine years of age.

People with lazy eye may also experience the following symptoms: poor depth perception, head tilt, reduced vision in one eye. Conventional medicine treats amblyopia by having the patient wear a patch over the "good" eye, which requires the lazy eye to become aware of its surroundings. Prescription glasses or surgery may be used, or all may be used in combination.

Eye Movement Disorders

The area of functional conditions known as eye movement disorders is divided into three subsets:

1. Disorders of fixation, which have to do with the ability of the eyes to focus directly on a target without having to shift the eyes to somewhere else

2. Disorders of saccadic eye movements, which have to do with the ability to move the eyes from one area of space to another
3. Disorders of pursuit eye movements, which have to do with the ability to track a moving object with the eyes

Patients with ocular motor control problems may also experience the following symptoms: head turning as the eyes scan a line of printed words, the need to use a finger to target print, omission of small words in reading, poor attention span, difficulty with certain tasks, including driving, sports, reading, and writing.

Conventional medicine has no treatment for eye movement disorders, and the condition is often overlooked in examinations unless it is objectively apparent.

Refractive Problems

Refractive problems are those that involve the manner in which light is bent or shaped once it enters the eyes. Among the conditions in this category are astigmatism, farsightedness, nearsightedness, and presbyopia.

Astigmatism

The term *astigmatism* is taken from the Greek *a*, meaning "without," and *stigma*, meaning "point." A cornea that is football-shaped instead of perfectly round defines this condition. The lens of the eye may also be misshapen. This concept of "without a point" refers to the fact that in the astigmatic eye, light rays do not come into a single point of focus. Instead, light is distorted as it enters the eye and a blurred image forms on the retina. Astigmatism is very common and frequently occurs along with nearsightedness or farsightedness. When the condition occurs, it usually impacts both eyes, although it may be found in just one eye.

The person with astigmatism may also experience other symptoms, including blurred vision at near or far and at the tilt of the head.

Further, the person's eyes feel strained and may physically hurt when doing detail work. For people with astigmatism, straight lines may look crooked, and lines may be clearer in one direction over another. For example, horizontal lines may be clearer than vertical, or vice versa.

As with other functional conditions, astigmatism is not a fixed condition. A study of symphony musicians before and after the symphony season found profound changes in the amount of astigmatism in their prescriptions. These changes occurred because the musicians held their heads and eyes in a tilted position for hours at a time while playing concerts. In doing so, they offset the natural balance of eye muscles and created an artificial form of astigmatism.

The conventional treatment for astigmatism involves prescription lenses. In my office, however, I approach the problem differently. Such was the case when forty-seven-year-old Joan came to me for help. She had been wearing glasses for nearly forty years. When she came to me, her symptoms included a constant head tilt to the left and intermittent neck pain on the right. She told me that in the past ten years, the amount of her astigmatism and the angle of it had shifted four times. She had consistently asked her eye doctors why this was happening, but they had all told her the same thing: her eyes were misshapen.

Although her eyes were not perfectly shaped, I told her, that only accounted for part of her condition, most likely its onset. The changes in her astigmatic prescription in the last decade were due to the manner in which she used her eyes and the posture with which she held her head.

I then asked her to stand up and look directly ahead of her in a natural manner. When I asked if she were tilting her head at that moment, she said she wasn't. I straightened her head for her and she then reported that it felt tilted.

Together we planned her home-based program of vision therapy. In addition, I gave her a new prescription that reduced the amount of astigmatism in her glasses. I also showed Joan how to correctly set up her workstation at her place of employment to ensure that her head, neck, and torso were properly aligned.

After a few months of therapy, Joan's astigmatism had reduced by 50 percent and her neck pain had disappeared.

Hyperopia (Farsightedness)

The term *hyperopia* comes from the Greek *hyper*, meaning "far" or "over," and *opia*, meaning "eye." The hyperopic eye is also misshapen; the cornea is flatter than normal or the eye is of less than normal length, which causes the light rays that enter the eye to focus behind the retina instead of on it. People who are farsighted are able to clearly make out objects that are a long distance away, while near objects are more difficult to see.

Many children experience farsightedness without experiencing any problems of visual acuity. This is due to their greater ability to focus their eyes, which can compensate for the farsightedness.

Farsightedness can almost be considered the norm for newborns and young children. The farsightedness of those for whom it is a life-long condition may go unnoticed and untreated until they reach middle age, because until that time the eye's focusing mechanism was still able to compensate so that they saw normally.

Those who are farsighted may also experience the following symptoms: difficulty doing close work, especially reading; blurred vision; eyestrain; headaches; tension in the eyes. The only treatment conventional medicine has for farsightedness is prescription lenses.

Note that most of the world's population is farsighted; this makes sense historically. When our ancestors roamed the world, hunting for their day's food, they did not have to use their eyes to do sustained close work. Instead, they needed to see long distances in order to survive.

Today, only in such technological nations as the United States, Japan, England, and Germany is farsightedness *not* the norm. These cultures have different lifestyles, different work requirements and, therefore, different vision issues from those of other countries.

In the United States today, we are detail-oriented, and many times, the farsighted person in our culture has a harder time achieving in school. That may be one reason why a higher percentage of people with farsightedness are found to have learning disabilities.

Presbyopia (Middle-Aged Eyes)

The term *presbyopia* comes from two Greek words, *presby*, meaning "older," and *opia*, meaning "eye." It relates to the natural decrease of the eye's ability to focus as we age. This is due to a gradual stiffening of the lens of the eye. Onset of presbyopia is usually around age forty, growing worse over the next twenty years.

Those with presbyopia experience difficulty focusing clearly close-up. Referring to the normal reading distance, many say that their arm has suddenly grown too short.

While conventional medicine has nothing to offer except pre-scription glasses, my vision therapy has shown that people who daily perform simple focusing exercises experience a great benefit.

Such was the case with Barbara, a fifty-five-year-old exercise instructor who had worn reading glasses for a decade. As an advocate for physical exercise, she was determined to not let her eyes get any less active than any other part of her body. For Barbara, I put together a very simple home-based program of daily exercises. Three months later, when she next visited the office, an examination showed that she was able to see at near distances with half the prescription that she had needed only a few months ago. Over the months, Barbara was able to continue reducing her prescription, until she was finally able to read once more without glasses.

Myopia (Nearsightedness)

The term *myopia* comes from the Greek verb *myops*, which means "to close," and, again, *opia*, meaning "eye." Thus the term literally means "to close your eyes." In the United States, this is the most common functional eye condition.

The nearsighted are able to see near objects more clearly than objects that are farther away. Onset of the condition usually occurs between ages eight and twelve. It usually grows worse for a period of years before stabilizing in the late teens or early twenties. According to conventional thought, the tendency toward nearsightedness appears to be largely hereditary. Those who are nearsighted commonly experience the following symptoms: inability to see at a distance, the need to squint their eyes in order to see clearly, eyestrain.

Myopia tends to impact both eyes, although one may be worse than the other. Frequently diagnosed after a student is observed squinting while trying to read the blackboard, it is commonly treated with prescription glasses. Glasses bend the light entering the eyes to focus it correctly on the retina and relay a clear image to the brain.

More than eighty million people in the United States are myopic. In other words, we are faced with a literal epidemic of myopia in our nation. And yet, it seems to be an epidemic that the public is quite willing to accept.

Are we foolish enough to continue to think that the condition is merely inherited or is simply a natural part of our lives? This becomes especially improbable when we look at our own eyes compared with those of the rest of the world. We are a society of nearsighted people living in a farsighted world. And yet, nearsightedness is considered almost normal in the United States.

On an optical level, nearsightedness is easy to understand. Normally, light enters the eye, is bent by the cornea, then bent by the lens, and finally focused on the retina. In the myopic eye, the light is focused in front of the retina. This makes the image of distant objects blurred. In seeking to treat myopia, the eye doctor measures the amount of blur and prescribes a lens that bends the light so that it focuses on the retina and the image appears clear. A concave lens is used in the treatment of this disorder.

But how have so many Americans become nearsighted? Less than 5 percent of Americans are born myopic. Most become myopic during the first eighteen years of life. By ten years of age, only 10 percent are myopic; by fifteen, 25 percent; and by eighteen, fully 40 percent. (Those involved with higher education increase the numbers: 60 percent of college students are myopic, as are 75 percent of those in graduate school.)

I believe that the number of persons with myopia has more to do with our lifestyles and the way that we use our eyes than it does with genetics. It is no simple coincidence that the years of onset correspond with the years of schoolwork, book learning, and computer work.

Myopia is a prime example of what is called function affecting structure. The more we read and do computer work, the more time we spend locked in tasks involving near vision, the more difficult it becomes to see distance. Book learning involves tightening the ciliary muscles to see near, and the longer these muscles are tightened, the more difficult it becomes to relax them when the task is completed. Further, this tightening of the ciliary muscle around the lens over time actually causes the eyeball to lengthen, creating an artificial but quite permanent myopic state.

Many studies over the years have borne out this theory. A particularly telling one involved 140 Native Alaskan children. When first tested, only two children in that pool showed signs of myopia. These children continued to be tracked and tested over the next thirty years as American schools were introduced into the culture. Over those years, the cases of myopia increased until some 35 percent of the children tested as nearsighted. Yet their parents and grandparents who escaped schooling still tested at less than 5 percent myopic.

The ways we use our eyes have created this terrible epidemic. Yet conventional eye care doctors are quite happy to just hand out more glasses. Over time and as their patients' eyes get more myopic, doctors prescribe stronger glasses. There is nothing done about the cause of the condition or to improve the patients' eyes.

In my office, I approach myopia differently. Such was the case with Samantha, an eight-year-old third-grader. Samantha was very smart, very quick, and a perfectionist. She had little interest in sports or other activities but was very motivated in her schoolwork and loved to read.

When I tested Samantha, she had only 20/100 distance visual acuity in both eyes. She had worn glasses for a year but had recently failed the school's vision test. Her mother was worried because she herself was very myopic and she wanted her daughter to have better eyes than she had.

I strongly recommended that Samantha undergo a course of vision therapy, both at home and in my office, that would stress relaxation and natural vision enhancement. I placed the emphasis on what I call "visual hygiene," an approach that teaches patients to properly treat their eyes, just as they already do the other parts of the body. Samantha was also strictly regulated on the amount of close work she could do before taking a break and resting her eyes. I also prescribed a special pair of bifocal glasses for Samantha, which she was to wear while in the classroom. She could look through the top part of the glasses to see the teacher and the blackboard and use the bottom part for her reading and close work.

Even with vision therapy, Samantha's myopia continued to worsen for a time before it stabilized and began to improve.

You may have noticed by this time that, for each category of functional conditions, conventional medicine offers only prescription glasses—or worse, surgery—in terms of treatment. And while glasses may sometimes be necessary, you need not accept treatment of your functional condition that is merely a physical crutch. At best, this will only hold the condition in check. At worst, it will worsen your condition and possibly your overall health.

In the chapters to come, I will discuss the underlying causes of these conditions and potential alternative treatments. But let us first turn our attention to other eye ailments—the pathological conditions.

Pathological Conditions

There are far too many disease states of the eyes to list them all here. But four conditions are far more common and will be considered in the pages that follow: cataracts, dry eyes, glaucoma, and macular degeneration.

Cataracts

Perhaps cataracts can best be described as opaque spots on the lens of the eye. These spots block sufferers' vision, and at best, they see as if through a cloud or a haze. These spots can vary in size, density, and location on the eye. Therefore, their impact on vision can vary. Many people notice the onset of cataracts when they require more light for reading and have difficulty reading street signs as they drive. They may also experience difficulties with depth perception. This can be particularly problematic with the elderly, for whom failing depth perception may cause falls and accidents, resulting in serious injury.

Cataracts will grow worse over time. They are said to "ripen," growing larger and/or denser. They are the major cause of blindness. In the United States alone, some 40 million people suffer from cataracts. In recent years, removal of cataracts has become the single most common surgical procedure covered by Medicare, with some 600,000 surgeries done annually.

Age is an important factor for cataracts. Only some 15 percent of the population is afflicted with cataracts before age 55, but the figure jumps to 50 percent by age 75, and up to 90 percent by age 85.

Note that of all eye diseases, cataracts are the most responsive to conventional medical treatments. The standard treatment is to remove the lens through a method called *phacoemulsification*. In this treatment, a surgeon uses an ultrasonic beam to break up the hardened lens and then vacuums up the pieces with a suction device. He or she then replaces the cataracted lens with an artificial lens, called an intraocular lens (IOL).

The procedure has become both quick and easy, and I recommend it now for my patients who are experiencing severe vision loss due to cataracts, although I also make a point of having my patients understand that cataracts do not need to be a part of the natural aging process. They are, rather, the result of an underlying condition and a sign that the natural processes of the body are breaking down. Normal flows of nutrients to the eyes have been compromised, as have the flow of waste products back out of the eyes. If the underlying problem is left untreated, conditions even worse than cataracts may occur.

Even those who choose to undergo cataract surgery should seek to improve their overall health before the invasive procedure. Because cataracts develop slowly over a period of years, there is usually time for preventive measures to be very successful. If the condition is identified early on, surgery may be avoided. Nutritional counseling is often very helpful, as are other forms of alternative medicine. Dietary additives including vitamin C, alpha lipoic acid, and lutein have all been shown to have merit in the prevention of cataracts. It is also important for everyone to protect their eyes by wearing sunglasses that block 100 percent of UVA and UVB light.

Dry Eyes

Dry eyes is probably the single most common complaint that patients bring to their eye doctors. Technically known as aqueous insufficiency, dry eyes affects more than thirty-three million Americans. People in all age groups complain that their eyes feel dry. They also say that their eyes feel gritty, irritated, and burn or alternate between dryness and watering.

Any condition that reduces the production or composition of tears can result in dry eyes. Like most pathological conditions, dry eye syndrome is often related to health issues tied to other parts of the body. Most often, it is associated with a general dryness of the mucous membranes. It may also be related to brittle joints and nails.

Dry eyes are much more common in women than in men. Research suggests that fluctuations in hormone levels, particularly estrogen and the androgens, may result in dry eye syndrome. Pregnant women, women taking birth control pills, and postmenopausal women who take hormone replacement therapy all report dry eyes.

Dry eyes in postmenopausal women may be a sign of Sjogren's syndrome. This condition affects up to four million American women and may be the most commonly misdiagnosed condition in women over age forty. Those suffering from Sjogren's syndrome often experience dryness throughout their system, with dry eyes, dry and cracked lips, dry scalp, and brittle nails. The syndrome is caused when a breakdown occurs in the autoimmune system and antibodies actually attack fluid-secreting cells in the body. Other symptoms of the syndrome include a general feeling of fatigue and a tendency toward cavities in the teeth.

As with other conditions, age tends to be a factor in dry eye syndrome. Older patients have a greater tendency toward dry eyes. In fact, as we get older, our eyes produce up to 40 percent less lubrication naturally.

Long-term contact lens use can also contribute to dry eyes, as, over time, contact lenses lessen corneal sensitivity. The sensitivity of the cornea determines how many tears will be secreted.

Cigarette smoke is also a huge contributing factor. Up to 40 percent of those with dry eyes are either smokers or people who live or work in a smoke-filled atmosphere. Other environmental factors that contribute to dry eyes include air-conditioning, environmental allergens, and wind. Many medicines can also produce dry eyes, especially antihistamines, diuretics, and oral contraceptives.

Ironically, the over-the-counter eye drops that millions buy to help alleviate dry eyes may actually cause their eyes to get drier still. While these drops may bring temporary relief, they have nothing more than a palliative effect. The preservatives in the drops will, in the long run, actually make the condition worse. Long-term use may, in fact, kill corneal cells. Eye drops that contain vasoconstrictors—those that act to take the redness out of the eye—actually reduce the blood circulation in the eye and decrease the production of tears, making the eyes drier still.

If you choose to use eye drops, make sure to use only those without preservatives, such as Viva drops from Vision Pharmaceuticals or Thera Tears from Advanced Vision Research. These can actually enhance corneal healing and the production of tears. New brands of drops on the market today also have antioxidants and vitamin A added. These are especially healing to the eyes.

For a more permanent form of relief, conventional medicine offers punctal occlusion, a medical procedure by which the drain that draws away excess fluids from the eyes is actually closed. While some eye care professionals may feel it is an effective treatment for the problem of dry eyes, I consider its use only in the most difficult cases. It certainly should not be undertaken lightly, and alternative treatments should be considered first.

Glaucoma

Glaucoma, or "chronic open angle," is an insidious eye disease that can be difficult to detect until a significant amount of vision is already lost. The reason it can be such a dangerous condition is because those suffering from this disease experience no symptoms at all, feel no pain, and maintain 20/20 vision. Yet, if left undetected, glaucoma can slowly steal peripheral vision until sufferers feel as if they are peering through a tunnel—at best. Very often, 70 percent of the vision is already gone by the time the condition is diagnosed.

As many as fifteen million Americans have chronic glaucoma—although only about half that many are ever actually diagnosed with the disease. Of those, nearly two million have already experienced vision loss, and more than a quarter of a million are blind in one eye. Glaucoma costs sufferers more than two and a half billion dollars a year in treatments, and these numbers are rising as the baby boomers move through middle age.

What is glaucoma? Technically, it is caused by damage to the optic nerve itself, often as a result of increased pressure in the aqueous humor, the clear watery fluid that circulates in the chamber of the eye between the cornea and the lens. However, it can occur even with normal intraocular pressure.

In a healthy eye, aqueous humor is produced and then drained from the eye into the bloodstream at a constant rate, so that there is always a fresh supply and steady amount. The draining of the aqueous humor occurs through a small canal located between the iris and the cornea.

In some cases, too much aqueous humor begins to be produced and the eye cannot express it quickly enough. This causes a buildup from what is called normal intraocular pressure. In other cases, the correct amount of humor is created, but a blockage occurs in the drainage system. In either case, the abnormally high pressure that results is called *intraocular hypertension*. It is this increased pressure that damages the ocular nerve. At first, the peripheral vision is affected and the central vision—the sight of objects directly in front of the eyes—is left unaffected. As the condition develops, more and more of the central vision is affected, until blindness finally results.

Parts of the population are harder hit than others: Hispanic Americans have twenty times the risk of developing the disease than do Caucasians. African Americans have four times the risk until age forty-five, at which time the likelihood increases to seventeen times that of whites.

Contributing factors include obesity and arthritis. While hypertension, or high blood pressure, has not yet been found to be a direct factor, studies have shown it to be statistically related to glaucoma.

At present, conventional treatment for glaucoma is either allopathic medication or surgery.

Macular Degeneration

Macular degeneration is the slow, steady deterioration of the cells of the *macula*, the tiny yellowish area near the center of the retina, the area of the eye where vision is most acute. Macular degeneration causes deterioration of the central vision, the vision that is used for reading, writing, and driving. Those with macular degeneration perceive straight lines as crooked, distinct shapes as blurry, and a patch of fog at the center of the visual field. Where the glaucoma sufferers experience a loss of vision from the outside of the vision field inward toward the center, macular degeneration sufferers experience vision loss from the center outward. As with glaucoma, macular degeneration can lead to blindness.

There are two types of macular degeneration. Some 90 percent of those with the disease suffer from what is called *dry macular degeneration*. In this dry type, small yellow spots called *drusen* form underneath the macula. These drusen slowly break down the cells of the macula, distorting the vision. Dry macular degeneration can advance to the second, more serious form of the disease, which is called *wet macular degeneration*.

In wet macular degeneration, new and abnormal blood vessels begin to grow toward the macula. These new vessels leak blood and fluid, which further degenerates the macula, causing rapid and severe loss of vision.

At the present, there is no treatment for macular degeneration, although laser surgery has been used in severe cases. The attempt is to seal the leaks in the blood vessels, without permanently damaging the nerve fibers that travel through the same area.

As with glaucoma, the best treatment for macular degeneration is prevention, which, in this case, is largely tied to diet. Including the proper nutrients in the diet goes a long way toward assuring that the eyes are nourished as well.

CHAPTER 5

Vision and Adaptation

The Causes of Common Vision Impairments

"My mind is trying to tell me something through my eyes!"
—An anonymous patient

Before I begin discussing the causes of common vision disorders, it is important to note that our eyes are our means of reaching out to the world, as well as the way we receive information from the farthest point. Certainly our twenty-or-so feet of visual arena is a space far greater than we can reach with our hands. Likewise, it is a greater space than we can attain by the means of any other sensory input.

For a given person to be able to see and understand clearly what she has seen is as dependent upon parental bonding and societal development as it is upon physical growth. When vision skills are fully and completely developed, the environment actually becomes an extension of that individual, so that her awareness of it is the same as her awareness of her own body. At the same time, she can clearly distinguish between the two.

If, however, the eyes are traumatized through the use of improper medication, disease, or physical or emotional impact, vision is interfered with and comprehension fails to develop.

The human mind is an amazingly complex organ that is the site of consciousness. Often, when trauma of any sort occurs, the mind will begin to adapt to the trauma, even if it is not capable of healing it. The traumatized individual begins to make adaptations around the trauma and to develop ways of seeing and comprehending. While these adaptations do not represent the quintessence of vision, they do represent that individual's best attempt at attaining balance.

The last chapter discussed the ways in which vision can develop in a less-than-perfect manner, common functional and pathological conditions of the eye. Now I will discuss the underlying themes of these conditions and the adaptations they specifically suggest.

Themes and Adaptations in Functional Conditions

Binocular Disorders

Remember, our eyes are not a single organ but are instead two separate organs that have to function in concert in order for us to see clearly and correctly. How many relationships do you know of in which both partners get along at all times? Many vision conditions can be seen as a breakdown in the relationship between two beings.

With that idea in mind, let's consider again the common binocular disorders to which eyes are commonly vulnerable.

When I have considered the inability of one of my patient's two eyes to work together, I have to deal with a chicken-or-the-egg situation. I ask myself if a problem in the patient's mind is causing his eyes to function poorly or a problem with the patient's eye is causing his mind to misunderstand the image sent. Now, into this mix I must add a third possibility: maybe environmental and lifestyle stresses have placed such demands upon his visual system—his eyes and his brain— that they were just not designed to handle, causing a breakdown in his visual system.

Time and again, I have observed that when my patients have issues with binocularity they tend to also display certain characteristics. They will have difficulty physically and mentally staying in a situation in which there is a great deal of visual stimuli, such as a crowded train station or movie theater. These situations will cause a great deal of anxiety for those with issues of binocularity, as they have trouble integrating all the information that is being absorbed by their two eyes. They also tend to have issues with motion, especially the mechanical motions involved with travel. They tend to get car sick very easily. They are unable to read while in a moving vehicle.

Convergence Excess

Typically those with issues of convergence excess like to physically get very close to the person to whom they are speaking. In the same way, they tend to be very demanding in relationships and need their relationships to be very intimate.

Those with the tendency to overconverge with their eyes tend also to have a fear of losing control. As an adaptation they tend to suppress this fear—indeed, they may suppress *all* fear—and overwork with both their eyes and their mind. They tend to try too hard to succeed in all that they undertake and often do entirely too much—usually to the detriment of their eyes and their physical and emotional beings. This condition can lead to eyestrain, headaches, and, very often, to nearsightedness.

Those who live and work with overconvergers report that they can be very controlling and are strong perfectionists.

Convergence Insufficiency

Sufferers of convergence insufficiency have an invisible force field around them, keeping people at a distance. They tend to stand back or back away as they speak to other people. When dealing with patients with convergence insufficiency, I try to be very careful to keep a comfortable distance from them so that they will not begin to feel stress.

In my clinical experience, the inability of a patient to converge her eyes usually indicates low willpower. This patient's core issue tends to be a certain degree of hopelessness and a lack of personal vital force. She tends to go through life either in a state of vague anxiety or motivated directly by fear. Fear and anxiety paralyze her as she approaches the world and her life in it. She is easily overwhelmed. Every effort, especially a new undertaking, seems to be too much for her.

Strabismus

The patients with strabismus who have come into my office range between three and seventy-five years old. Some have been spared the operations that are supposed to correct the condition. Others have had as many as four operations without the hoped-for result. The goal of the operation is to make the person's eyes look normal. It is not the primary goal of the operation to help the eyes work as a team. If that occurs at all, it is a secondary result.

Over 80 percent of the patients I have seen with strabismus do not have adequate binocularity in their eyes for them to function fully. This can be true even if their eyes appear straight to others.

So what is the underlying cause of this condition? Is it just a muscular condition, as allopathic medicine would insist, or is it a fundamental breakdown in the eye-brain connection? Using my own patients as a living laboratory, I have explored both the reasons for and the nature of strabismus.

I have found that strabismus suddenly occurs when there is great stress in the environment, especially in a child's environment. A young child may suddenly exhibit eye turn when there is a death in the family or when his parents announce that they plan to divorce. In my opinion, this is the child's way of saying, "I don't want to deal with the world anymore," after he feels that someone he loved has failed or deserted him. It is also his way of saying that he can no longer deal completely with all that is going on in his world.

When I explore the underlying emotional component of the condition with my patients, I find that a common theme among them is the feeling that they are not complete, that something is missing within them. Many feel ill at ease in social settings and lack self-esteem. Certainly, most also feel a sense of embarrassment concerning how their eyes look. Both this embarrassment and their general sense of social inadequacy lead them to withdraw from the world.

What is so exciting about working with these particular patients is that as their eyes begin to naturally straighten through vision work, many of their personality issues—especially that lack of self-esteem—dramatically improve. For many patients with strabismus, I find it necessary to strongly suggest that they use psychotherapy as an adjunct to vision therapy. Doing both seems to greatly enhance both their physical and emotional recovery.

Note that in my clinical experience, even those patients with strabismus who have no visible symptoms of eye turn still display the same personality issues—perhaps to a lesser degree—than do those with a visible turn. As they use their dual therapies as tools to recovery, that recovery is equally dramatic.

Esotropia

The underlying message of an inward-turning eye is "I have to protect myself." For me, that inward turn is like a turtle going into its shell.

Much like their eyes, the bodies of patients with esotropia tend to go into a protective posture and turn inward to protect themselves. I have observed that their eye turns also manifest in other parts of the body. Some also have feet that turn inward. Others tend to turn one or both shoulders inward. But all are in a state of constant alert and self-protection.

I invariably find in my practice that the esotropes tend to exhibit a profound lack of flexibility, both in body and in spirit. They lock into emotional, physical, and spiritual patterns, patterns again based in self-protection. They use a great deal of their energy keeping other people out.

Exotropia

In my experience, when a person's eye turns out, she is saying, "Only half of me is really here. I can look at you, talk with you, but I am not really present here with you." It is as if she experiences the world as a daydream.

Where esotropes turn inward in a protective stance, exotropes tend to shut down a part of themselves as a means of protection and coherence. (In terms of their physical posture, I have found that they tend to wear out the outside edges of their shoes because they put their weight on the outside of their feet.)

If exotropes—or esotropes, for that matter—are aware through both of their eyes at once, they will experience double vision. Therefore, most exotropes will shut down and suppress the image of one of their eyes. Since this a survival adaptation and does not have a physical cause, this suppression cannot be corrected with lenses. The suppression actually makes the exotrope better able to deal with the conflicting images that each eye is presenting.

The core emotion most common to exotropes is a feeling of a lack of safety. They will spend a great deal of their energy trying to create a situation in which they can feel physically and emotionally secure. Their spirits yearn to feel nurtured. To attain this they shut down a portion of their being and feel emotionally numb. Exotropes also live in denial of the physical fact that they have two eyes. One of my goals for their vision therapy is to get the two eyes to act as partners and allow them to attain a level of inner peace.

Amblyopia

Amblyopia is often defined as a condition where the acuity of an eye is reduced, and that reduction is not correctable through optical means.

Obviously, this condition can be related both to exotropia and to esotropia, as presented above. But it need not be associated with the turning of an eye. There can be other reasons why a person might suppress the vision from an eye.

Those reasons almost always have to do with the failure of other vision skills. Amblyopia usually accompanies binocular disorder like exotropia and poor binocular skills like poor focusing ability (wherein one eye may have a much greater degree of nearsightedness than the other), poor eye movement control, poor eye-hand coordination (although this may be the product of amblyopia as well as its cause), and poor ability to process visual information from the eye.

No matter the specific cause of the lazy eye, the underlying issue remains the same: trust. The person cannot trust the information that is taken in from one eye. Because of this, he comes to have issues of trust with everything in his world, including his relationships.

I have asked my patients to patch their "good," or dominant, eye and then to look at their lazy eye in a mirror. When I then ask them how they feel, they report that they are uncomfortable. "I don't like to use this eye," they say. "It feels old and lazy."

When, through the process of natural vision improvement, I prove to them that that eye has more ability than they believed, the patients respond with almost a miraculous increase in vision in the affected eye. What once was a dull and "lazy" eye, an object of shame, becomes a vital organ.

In no other aspect of my practice do I see the relationship between the eyes and the mind as clearly as I do when working with an amblyope. In many cases, as they come to trust the information taken in from the lazy eye, their whole belief system shifts and they become able to trust their world and all that's in it.

I received the following letter after I had published a book of Magic Eye 3-D images. To me, it illustrates the power of the mind in relation to amblyopia.

> All my life, I've had one eye that was significantly weaker than the other. When I was twenty-eight years old, an optometrist tested me and told me my weaker eye was essentially turned off and that I had no binocular depth perception. The doctor also told me that there was nothing to correct my condition.
>
> After working with the 3-D pictures, I can now see the depth in the pictures. But even more incredible is the fact that my every-day, real-world vision has changed. I now see with both my eyes all the time.

> The only way this could be more exciting would be if I had been
> blind all my life and woke up one day able to see.

Perhaps the underlying issue here is one of neglect. Some part of the amblyope feels that it has not been nourished as it should have been and feels, perhaps, unloved. That may be why vision therapy targeted on restimulating the weakened eye can so miraculously turn the condition around.

Many times I have found that as the lazy eye becomes active, a multitude of negative emotions is aroused. Amblyopes may feel anger, frustration, fear, or sorrow as their eye begins to see. This is one of the groups for whom I tend to keep a good deal of Kleenex on hand.

Eye Movement Disorders

Disorders of eye movement have underlying themes as well. In general, regarding all issues of eye movement, I have come to understand that there is an uncontrolled aspect of energy in patients. This uncontrolled energy is often most obvious in their behavior; they are excited, enthusiastic, and sometimes even manic.

This adaptation seems to be highly verbal as well. Sufferers tend to lack adequate skills to edit their own speech and invariably say things they don't mean. This outpouring of energy, both in manic behavior, and, worse, in trying to reign in that behavior, leaves these people feeling chronically exhausted and depressed.

The other underlying reason for this adaptation is quite the opposite: the energy of those with disorders of eye movement is blocked or totally deficient, and they may be extremely sad. They are given to long-term melancholy and at their core tend to feel that they are both unlovable and unloved.

Eye movement skills allow us to obtain the greatest amount of information in the shortest amount of time with the least amount of effort. To function correctly, the eyes must be able to scan space with speed and control.

If we remember that vision comes not from the eye but from the brain, then it should come as no surprise that those who have issues with uncontrolled eye movements also have trouble focusing their minds. For this reason, a high percentage of children and adults with attention deficit disorder (ADD) also have issues with their eye movement skills. As I explain to my patients, "Your eyes are going at one speed and your mind at another."

Therefore, as I work with such patients to increase their awareness and ability to monitor and control themselves, I find that they develop an ability to control their eye movements. As that control develops, their depression lifts, and they find themselves with energy sufficient to finish all necessary tasks.

Refractive Problems

In treating patients with refractive problems I have quite often found that the underlying issues involved are those of time and space.

Astigmatism
People with astigmatism often experience the world as a painful and exhausting place. The astigmatic person has, at some critical point in her life, received a mixed message. Perhaps the support received from one parent was undermined by the other, or perhaps parents and teachers disagreed about her basic value as a human being. Somewhere the astigmatism sufferer has been fundamentally confused by the information she has received. The outward distortion of the world that she has received through her eye condition is basically a mirror of the distortion of her inner self.

Hyperopia
The farsighted patients that come into my office are there for several different reasons, mainly their inability to focus on close work. The symptoms that surround that issue can be as varied as eyestrain, exhaustion, blurring of vision, and the inability to read for more than the

briefest periods of time. By the time they come into my office, the symptoms have been in place for a long time.

Most farsighted people are farsighted from birth, and their adaptations to the condition have been in place for many years before I see them. Because of this, it can be difficult to reformat the adaptation to a healthier way of seeing.

Even though the condition does not arise from a specific trauma, there is a behavioral component to hyperopia, a strategy for dealing with the world that tends to underlie sufferers' specific symptoms. Most are extroverted, have a great desire to know what others are thinking, and want to make a connection in the world, to contact others.

They are also active people. Farsighted people are natural hunter-gatherers who, in today's world, often put those skills to use in playing sports. These are not people who would be likely to sit for hours staring at a chessboard.

Hyperopes love change and dislike a daily routine. They don't enjoy a desk job in a cubicle that offers stability and a regular paycheck. Nor do they want to spend long hours in class, followed by hours of reading and worrying about details like mathematical sums and historical dates. They may receive grades far below those that they could achieve and may also be considered as having behavior problems since they naturally chafe against having to spend the whole day trapped in a classroom behind a small desk. The fact that they are not natural or happy students does not mean they lack intelligence, but it does mean that they tend to show their intelligence in ways other than book learning.

Hyperopes may, in fact, have some trouble remembering the past or staying in the present, as they are frequently future-oriented.

In my practice I have found that hyperopia, like any number of other vision disorders, is not a fixed condition. A patient's degree of farsightedness can vary greatly due to a number of factors, chief among them the amount of stress under which the patient is placed and the amount of detail work he is required to undertake.

If I can convince the farsighted patient that I am trying to work with him through issues that have proven to be both most painful and most boring, then there is an excellent chance that I can bring his condition to normal, depending upon the degree of hyperopia that he was born with. But because hyperopes have spent their entire lives trying to avoid details, vision therapy offers them possible fatigue and boredom and potential physical pain, as their eyes are exercised inward.

I must report that I have had many failures in working with hyperopes in my office, not because vision therapy techniques will not work with hyperopes, but because hyperopes will not work with vision therapy techniques. As future-oriented hunter-gatherers, they no more want to spend time staring at exercise cards and machines than they want to spend it reading and studying. For this reason, the majority of hyperopes who attend vision therapy in my office have been ordered to do so by the local school system.

Myopia

The vision therapy for myopes is quite different from that of other problems. I feel joy when I hear the sigh that issues from the myope whose eyes have just been relaxed through vision therapy. Where some patients, like the amblyopes, cry from sorrow and others, the hyperopes, cry in pain (the exercises give them a headache), the myopes tend to fill the room with laughter as they experience a sensation of lightness and freedom that they often have not known before. For the first time in their life, their eyes are relaxed and their minds are at peace.

Unlike hyperopia, most people with myopia are not born with it. Most, however, develop myopia either by the way society demands that they use their eyes or as a result of deep emotional and spiritual issues.

Underlying the condition of myopia are three main issues.

The first underlying issue is a weak or underdeveloped sense of self and/or an insufficient vital force. Such myopes are unsure of their own identities and of their paths in life. Often, they will also be unsure of their own opinions, so that they will turn to others in order to find out what they should be thinking and doing. These people usually have weak boundaries and may be psychically unaware of just where their energy ends and others' begins. Such myopes tend to be timid, to lack confidence, and to be plagued with self-doubt.

The second issue is deep feelings of insecurity, although the myope may seem energetic and forceful. To overcompensate for this feeling of uncertainty, such myopes become overly decisive and often act irritable and impatient with others. In other words, with this type, appearance is everything, and they work hard to appear to be in charge and in control. They put a great deal of store in the opinions of others, and it is important to them that others feel as if they have a solid grasp on their own life's path.

Most such myopes are overcompensating; few actually have a solid core. Those who do will be intolerant of others who are less sure, less quick, and they will tend to work to the betterment of their own ego, no matter the cost to others. These myopes will experience ongoing feelings of impatience, frustration, and depression as they move through life. Often, they will feel as if they were being blocked in every direction by the circumstances of their life.

Finally, the third underlying issue is a complex internal world of thoughts and worries that the myopes cannot translate into action and feel helpless to change. These myopes are deep worriers, people who may experience no emotion other than worry and anxiety. They will not be able to feel or bear intense feelings. On top of this, they tend to experience an ongoing sense of emptiness in their lives.

Some of these myopes have deeper issues and troubles. Some exhibit obsessive-compulsive behaviors. Others are schizophrenics. A common factor is the feeling that they are not fully inhabiting their physical body or the physical world, although they worry endlessly about their health and their safety in the world.

No matter what the underlying issue, myopes will usually have issues of insecurity. The adaptation that they most often take to combat this insecurity is trying to please. If they feel they are failing to please another, they will simply try harder, work harder, strain more. They do this because of the way they perceive time.

Just as hyperopes are future-oriented to the point that they can almost completely forget that they have lived in the past, myopes are past-oriented. Often, they are mired completely in the past. You will find this in their emotional patterns, as they try again and again to dredge up old hurts and old emotions—both good and bad. Myopes remember every negative word that ever was said to them, and it is as if they had only been said moments ago. They also, however, clearly remember moments of joy and intimacy, moments that they try to create again and again, using the same old patterns and props with new people. They are always mystified when the moment of joy does not reoccur. It may be said that myopes spend so much time reliving their past lives that they are all but incapable of living the present ones.

Over 70 percent of all the patients who come to see me are myopic. They come in all different sizes and shapes: tall, short, heavy, thin. Some never wear glasses, although they need them, and others never take their glasses off. The conventional treatment for all of them is the same: just give them corrective lenses so that they can see things at a distance—case closed.

But how can this same treatment be effective for all of these individuals? Some of them became nearsighted at a very young age, while others didn't have any issue with myopia until they were in college.

As I said in the last chapter, this epidemic of myopia has a great deal to do with how we are using our eyes, especially with our link to computers. But it also has something to do with a deeper issue: how we are living our lives, how we are treating our eyes, and how they reflect all that is going on inside of us. More than any other eye condition, myopia reveals how we as Americans typically relate to the world around us.

I have been questioning my patients about their nearsightedness for more than twenty years, and in looking over the answers, I have started to see themes having to do with how they were looking at and dealing with the world at the time of the onset of their myopia. I have found that one to two years before they received their first glasses and within months of having to receive stronger glasses, the majority of my patients reported that they had one or more periods of feeling deeply inadequate and shy. They tended to withdraw from the world, to use their minds in an analytical manner, and to be drawn toward sedentary and intellectual pursuits, especially reading and computer activities. Further, they felt that their circumstances required them to keep their emotions to themselves. If there was a direct conflict in their life at that time—a divorce, for instance—they felt that circumstances required that they withdraw from that issue rather than confront it. Further, they sought positive reinforcement by trying to please others, often specifically trying to please the individual who was the greatest cause of their distress. In these people, there is a strong need to be "good" and to succeed in work, school, and the home.

On an optical level, nearsightedness may be said to be a way of cutting themselves off from the world by blurring it into a fog. They conclude, on some profoundly deep level, that they do not know how to deal with the world. They feel safer when they focus their analytical skills inward. Finally, they conclude that emotions cause pain and intellectual pursuits bring rewards, so they will feel less and think more.

Thus, in vision therapy, myopic patients are mired in the past and trapped in a small shell. Further, they are accustomed to not feeling things at all or to ignoring what they are feeling.

At first, some myopes are scared and feel very, very small and fragile. But many find themselves suddenly opening up again where they have closed down. When I provide them with the correct balance of clarity and blur, they become very, very happy.

Presbyopia

Most conventional doctors agree that there is something inevitable about presbyopia. As people age, their eyes age with them, and as part of that aging process, the eyes will lose their ability to focus easily. At some point everyone's arms get too short for them to be able to read easily.

Some people develop presbyopia in their early thirties. Others don't experience it until well into their fifties. Most, however, see changes in their vision when they are between forty-two and forty-five years of age.

Something in me, however, refuses to see the symptoms associated with presbyopia as natural or acceptable, so I turned again to my "living lab"—my patients—for the answer. I found a pattern in the personality traits of those experiencing the onset of presbyopia.

As middle-aged people become increasingly dissatisfied with their lives, they are more likely to notice a deterioration of their vision. The more they try new things as a way of patching and covering that dissatisfaction, the more their ability to focus on near vision deteriorates.

When I ask such patients to focus on what is happening to them at the moment and the more they try to clear up the actual issues rather than run from them or ignore them, the more their vision improves. After solving their issues and clearing their vision, they are then free to move on to new things in their life with joy and satisfaction.

In fact, I find that presbyopia is one of the most treatable of all vision conditions. While those who use conventional treatments would consider presbyopia incurable—or worse, not even a condition in need of help—my success rate slowing down the deterioration in this condition has been very high.

Themes and Adaptations in Pathological Conditions

While functional conditions may be caused by emotional or spiritual distress, it is easy to think that pathological conditions—those involving literal disease states—cannot be so easily dismissed. However, this is not the case. In my years of practice, I have consistently witnessed that our physical being literally shapes itself around our spiritual perception of ourselves. Therefore, while it would be easy to say that pathological eye conditions are someone or something else's fault (for example, that we caught glaucoma like a common cold), this is not the case.

I'm convinced that there are reasons why we develop the eye pathologies we do and that by treating them holistically and correctly, we can bring about a total healing.

Cataracts

Patients with cataracts have a cloudiness and uncertainty of inner vision. They tend to fear looking out into the world. In this way, I consider cataracts to be similar in adaptation to myopia; those suffering from them are of a similar emotional and spiritual state.

I have found cataract patients' nutritional biochemistry lacks specific nutrients, especially vitamin C and glutathione. Therefore, those with cataracts must establish and follow an overall nutritional program, whether or not they will undergo cataract surgery.

Kathy, a forty-eight-year-old woman who came into my office with the symptoms of moderate myopia, experienced slightly worse nearsightedness in her left eye than in her right. Otherwise, she was in excellent physical shape, doing yoga three times a week and exercising regularly.

Soon after she first came to my office, she complained that she was not able to see well at all through her right eye. After examining her, I noted that this eye exhibited the cloudiness associated with the early onset of a cataract.

I suspected that she may have recently experienced something traumatic in her life. She told me that she had recently left her husband after eighteen years of marriage. On top of that, her father was dying of cancer and she had decided to become his caregiver. I then discussed with her the meaning of the right eye as the male, or yang, eye and told her that issues with the vision in the right eye often corresponded to issues with the men in her life.

In traditional Chinese medicine, the right eye symbolizes the father, or all that is masculine in energy—goal-oriented, active, and assertive. Further, it symbolizes the process of logic, as it is located in the left side of the human brain. In traditional Chinese medicine, the left eye is considered the mother eye, representing all that is nurturing, receptive, and creative. In my experience in natural vision improvement, I have noticed again and again that those who have issues with their fathers or with the masculine principle itself will often manifest those issues as vision issues in their right eye. Mother issues manifest in the left eye.

Kathy and I decided that if she was to see well, she needed to deal with both her husband and her father in order to experience peace. We also agreed that she needed to begin psychotherapy in order to achieve this goal.

Within a year, Kathy returned to my office for a checkup, and we were both very happy to see that her cataract was gone.

Dry Eyes

Traditional Chinese medicine considers dry eyes to be the result of a deficiency in the kidney and liver meridians. This is because the flow of tears is controlled by the liver and because the kidneys play an important role whenever dryness is an issue in any part of the body.

On a purely physical level, dry eyes can also be caused by a nutritional imbalance. Spiritually, I believe dry eyes are a result of suppressing or hoarding grief. Often the people whose eyes are chronically dry have lost the ability to cry over the grief that they have experienced in their lives.

Scientific research has shown the presence of stress chemicals in human tears. It may therefore be concluded that a flow of tears is physically necessary in order to remove these chemicals from the system.

According to this research, the willingness to cry when under emotional pressure may actually prevent stress-related disease.

On the other hand, those who refuse to cry, who block grief and
pain in their lives rather than release it, will often develop chronically
dry eyes.

Glaucoma

In Chinese medicine, glaucoma is called liver energy stagnation
because the person who suffers from this malady may be said to have
shoved their negative emotions down deep inside over a period of years
until spiritual, emotional and, finally, physical energy builds.

It is certainly not news that our emotions affect the state of our
physical health and that stress makes glaucoma worse. As early as
1818, researchers linked glaucoma with stress. One study found that
a high percentage of glaucoma patients reported stressful life experiences at the time of the onset of their glaucoma. At times when the
patients' sense of security was most threatened, the pressure in their
eyes was greatly increased.

In addition to conventional medical treatment, I recommend
meditation, yoga, tai chi chuan, and/or psychotherapy for the patient
who suffers from glaucoma.

Macular Degeneration

I believe that macular degeneration is most common in those whose
life experience is clouded in sorrow. This condition will very often be
found in those who have lost a loved one, especially those who have
lost a loving husband or wife.

Sadly, a macular degeneration diagnosis or the experience of its
symptoms can actually make the condition itself worse. As sufferers
begin to lose their central vision, they become more and more afraid
that they will go blind. This fear causes internal stress, which causes

a lessening of circulation in the body and to the eyes, which then causes a worsening of the condition itself.

Meditation and relaxation techniques, therefore, can be helpful to those with macular degeneration, as can nutritional treatments that increase circulation. Lutein and bilberry are especially effective for those with macular degeneration.

Perhaps most important, however, is that those suffering from this condition need to involve themselves physically and emotionally with the world around them. They must be sure to spend time every week with others, in programs and groups, and not allow themselves to withdraw into a world of darkness and sorrow.

CHAPTER 6

Creating Better Vision

Options in Vision Care

"When I see, suddenly I am all eyes."
— Frederick Franck,
The Zen of Seeing

T hanks to ongoing advances in technology, the philosophy and practice of Western medicine is rapidly changing. The medical model of specialization—considering each specific symptom to be the domain of a particular specially trained physician—is being replaced by a model of wholeness, one that combines conventional treatments with complementary modalities of health care. Thus, the practice of eye care now involves a consideration of the patients' diet and exercise regimens, their relationships, and their lifestyle, in addition to the particular symptoms that brought them in for treatment in the first place.

As we move into the era of mind-body medicine, it becomes increasingly important that we understand our options in vision care and that we fully understand the differences among the myriad types of practitioners and therapies available. No form of medical practice is for everybody, and none will treat every form of illness effectively in everybody. But all offer valuable tools for healing.

Therefore, in this chapter I will discuss the nuts and bolts of vision care, both the practitioners and their unique forms of practice.

Choosing an Eye Doctor

Some of those who treat vision disorders are medical doctors and some are not. Some treat these disorders both with prescription lenses and with medications; others use only glasses. It is important that you understand the difference.

Ophthalmologist (M.D.)

An ophthalmologist is a medical doctor who specializes in diseases of the eye and in eye surgery. Ophthalmologists first attend college, where they take their prerequisite courses in science. They then attend medical school. After finishing both medical school and an internship, they enter a residency and fellowship training program to specialize in ophthalmology. This last stage in their training can last anywhere from three to eight years and focuses on the treatment of specific diseases of the eye with both medication and surgery. Thus ophthalmologists are allowed by law to diagnose diseases of the eye; to write prescriptions, both for medication and for prescription lenses; and to perform surgery on the eye.

Optometrist (O.D.)

Optometrists are primary health care providers who specialize in the examination, diagnosis, treatment, and management of diseases and disorders of the visual system—the eye and its associated structures— as well as the diagnosis of related systemic conditions. Optometrists must complete a four-year undergraduate program, taking prerequisite courses in chemistry, biology, physics, and mathematics. Then they must complete a second four-year program at a college of optometry. In optometry school, the training includes the diagnosis and treatment of eye disease and in how vision affects patients' performance in school, work, and sports. An important part of the training focuses on how patients use their eyes in their day-to-day life. Optometrists are taught to look for the functional causes of vision disorders. They are also taught how they can rehabilitate vision disorders through the use of lenses, prisms, and vision therapy. Note that though all optometrists are trained in vision therapy, only a small percentage of them offer this service as part of their practice.

Behavioral Optometrist (O.D.)

While they undergo the same education and training as a conventional optometrist, behavioral optometrists continue their education after the standard eight years in order to better understand the components of the human visual system. Behavioral optometrists may also be called developmental or functional optometrists. Behavioral vision care is based on the concept that vision is the dominant sense in humans and that it is a learned skill that begins to develop at the moment of birth, continuing throughout life. Behavioral optometrists use many different tools to help enhance patients' vision, from lenses, to posture work, to vision therapy. They stress the need for patients to understand how their lifestyle and use of their eyes impacts their quality of vision. (See Chapter 7 for more information on behavioral optometry.)

Optician

Opticians are trained to fill prescriptions that have been written by optometrists or ophthalmologists. They are taught how to make glasses and adjust eyeglass frames to a person's face. In some states, opticians are also allowed to fit contact lenses. They require only an associate's degree, which is usually a two-year program. Most states license opticians and require continuing education for them to retain that license.

Whatever category of eye care professional you choose, be sure to select one with whom you share a rapport. Does his office seem to be a safe place for you? Do you feel that you can confide in her all the personal information she might need in order to help you? Do you feel that along with your doctor you are a member of a team dedicated to your health and benefit?

Like going to the dentist, you may feel that the trip to the eye doctor is something of an ordeal, with many different machines being moved quickly in front of your face, many questions—"Which is clearer, this, or this?"—and an overall sensation of not having your needs met. Find the eye care professional whose personal philosophy of vision care best suits your own and whose style as a practitioner best fits your own style as a patient. If, for instance, you like to ask a lot of questions, find one who does not mind answering those questions. It sounds overly simple, but it is very important.

Remember, there are as many different ways to practice medicine as there are practitioners of medicine. No matter how well trained they may be, practitioners are just human beings. Never be afraid to ask questions on the telephone before making your first appointment. Ask about the doctor's education and his style of practice. Ask about the average length of his appointments and about the tools that he most often uses to improve vision. Ask if he practices vision therapy in his office or if he ever recommends vision therapy for his patients. Ask whether or not he is trained with any complementary forms of medicine in addition to his standard medical license.

In other words, do your research before you walk in the door. Know who the doctor is before he becomes your doctor. It takes a bit of time, but your needs will be better served in the long run by doing this bit of research.

It doesn't end on the telephone either. Your first appointment with an eye care professional is very important. During that appointment, if all goes well, you will clearly let the caretaker know what you expect of her and what your needs are as a patient, and she will let you know what her skills are as a practitioner. Hopefully, your needs and the doctor's skills will match, in which case you have the makings of a good doctor-patient team.

Finally, I believe eye contact is very important. Does your rapport with your eye doctor include solid eye contact as you exchange information? If you do not feel secure enough with your caretaker to look directly into his eyes as you talk, or, even worse, if he avoids direct eye contact, something is missing in the relationship.

The Tools of the Trade

Millions of people worldwide wear glasses or contact lenses, yet it is a pretty safe bet that few of them understand the principles by which either of these vision tools actually increase their ability to see clearly. Corrective lenses are by far the most common form of vision correction. Let's take a moment to consider what each involves.

Glasses

Basically, the lenses that are placed in front of the eyes bend light in a specific way so that the image that is carried through the eyes to the brain is clear and sharp. There are two basic types of lens, the *concave* lens, which is thinner in the middle than it is at the edge, and the *convex* lens, which is thinner on the edges and thickest in the middle.

The concave lens is also called the minus lens, because it decreases how much the light is bent, so that the light lands farther and farther back in the eye. This lens is used for nearsightedness, the condition in which the image focuses short of the back of the retina. With the appropriate lens, the image lands in the correct place. Therefore, those with nearsightedness will receive a prescription with a negative sign in front of a number to designate the strength of the prescription. The higher the number, the stronger the lens and the more light that has to be bent to make vision clear. Prescriptions between −0.25 and −1.50 are considered to treat mild degrees of nearsightedness; between −1.75 and −3.00, moderate nearsightedness; between −3.25 and −6.00; acute nearsightedness; over −6.00, severe nearsightedness.

The other type of lens, the convex, is used in the treatment of both farsightedness and presbyopia. (In presbyopia, the convex lens is used to increase the eye's focusing power, a power that age has lessened.) This lens is designated the plus lens, because it increases the amount of light that is bent in the eye, so that the light image lands forward in the eye. Again, the light is bent so that it lands directly on the retina and sends a sharp image to the brain.

With a convex lens, a prescription of up to +1.50 is considered a mild prescription; between +1.75 and +2.50, a moderate prescription; above +2.75, a potent prescription.

When glasses are used in the treatment of those with astigmatism, they are prescribed in a more complex manner. For those with astigmatism, the light taken into the eye focuses at two separate points in the eye. These points may both be in front of the retina, both behind it, or one in front and the other behind. The lens prescription given must bend light specifically so that it matches the particular curvatures of that eye and allows light to land in just the appropriate spot on the retina. This is called a cylindrical lens.

Millions of people today wear bifocals. This is a single pair of glasses with two different prescriptions. The prescription on the top of the lens is for distance seeing, and the prescription on the bottom is for near vision. Most of those who wear bifocals are older persons who, although nearsighted for many years, since middle age have developed issues with near vision as well. Thus they need prescriptions to help with both forms of vision.

Progressive lenses are sometimes used as an alternative to bifocals. They have more than the two prescriptions of bifocals and are often referred to as being multifocal lenses. With progressive lenses, the topmost section typically corrects for distance vision, the central part for intermediate vision, and the bottom part for near vision. They give the wearer a smooth transition from the distance portion of the lens to the reading portion.

Prism lenses are those where one side of the lens is thicker than the other. The purpose of the prism is to bend the light rays so that the eyes can function more effectively as a team. Thus, the patient who has an inward turn of an eye will wear a lens whose action is to bend the light to compensate for that turn. Prism glasses may make daily tasks like reading much easier for those with eye-teaming issues.

Contact Lenses

Contact lenses are used to correct such vision conditions as nearsightedness, farsightedness, astigmatism, and presbyopia. Sufferers of these conditions must undergo a thorough eye examination to determine whether or not they can wear contact lenses and which type of lens is best for them. While people of all ages can wear contact lenses, not all eyes are able to sustain wear. People with dry eyes tend to have trouble with contact lenses; even today's highly evolved ones cut off the flow of oxygen to the eyes. Some people's eyes are more sensitive than others to even the slightest oxygen depletion.

Still, the benefits of contact lenses are great. They increase peripheral vision and provide a more realistic image of an object. They eliminate the physical barrier between people and their worlds that is imposed by the use of glasses.

Allopathic Medications and Surgery

Allopathic medications and surgery are necessary for those people whose conditions cannot be controlled or corrected by the use of prescription lenses.

Such treatment is sometimes necessary and appropriate as a means of maintaining the gift of sight. Surgical treatment of eye disease is usually reserved for situations in which optical and medical treatment have failed or have been deemed inappropriate due to the nature of the condition. Surgery involves the use of either surgical instruments or lasers to physically alter the tissue in order to cure or correct an abnormality.

The most common form of surgery is *refractive surgery*, which is used to reshape the cornea, permanently changing the way light is bent in the eye so that the light focuses correctly on the retina. When performed correctly, refractive surgery can greatly reduce or totally eliminate a person's need for glasses or contact lenses.

Surgical eye treatments of any sort can and should only be performed by a qualified ophthalmologist. Note that surgery always has some risks associated with it and may often make rehabilitation of a vision condition more difficult.

Allopathic drugs are commonly used in the treatment of certain eye pathologies—for example, glaucoma and conjunctivitis—that cannot be corrected with lenses. While medications can be important and are sometimes necessary in halting the progress of eye disease, it is also important to correctly identify and treat the underlying cause of that disease. Also note that medications used to treat eye conditions can have side effects that impact sufferers' whole being.

Considering Complementary Therapies

In my more than twenty years' practice, I have often noticed that the holistic approach is the best and most effective approach to vision care. That is part of the reason why I chose to go back to school to get my degree in acupuncture and traditional Chinese medicine after I had already completed my training as a behavioral optometrist.

Over the years, I have referred patients to practitioners of complementary forms of medicine. This is not because I felt my own work inadequate but because I felt that if my patients could experience the healing potential of another modality in combination with my behavioral optometry, they could experience a healing, not just of their eyes, but of their whole beings.

The complementary forms of medicine that I most strongly recommend are discussed below.

Biofeedback Training

For years now, biofeedback has been used to measure and to regulate various bodily functions. In vision care, it is a powerful tool for the correction of refractive problems including myopia and hyperopia.

Joseph Trachtman, O.D., Ph.D., is the inventor of the Accommotrac vision trainer, which is the instrument that redefined biofeedback in terms of vision training. Here's how the instrument works. You look into the Accomotrac, and it measures the retina for clarity of image. As your focusing changes, the machine converts the visual image into a sound tone, so that very small changes of focus can be noticed and controlled. The treatment allows you to refine your control over your eye muscles, so whether you are nearsighted or farsighted you can significantly improve your vision.

The Accommotrac is often used in conjunction with vision therapy programs.

Syntonic Phototherapy

Syntonic phototherapy has been used clinically for more than sixty years. It represents a subset of the field of optometry in which vision disorders are treated through the application of selected visible light frequencies. A powerful adjunct to vision therapy, it has been shown to be helpful to those with strabismus, amblyopia, and eye-teaming issues. Syntonics is based upon the principle that certain frequencies (colors) or light shown through the eyes can restore balance to the body's regulatory centers, thereby affecting the core source of vision disorders.

Psychotherapy

Group or individual psychotherapy can be a helpful adjunct to vision treatment, especially when there are emotional issues at the core of an individual's vision disorders.

I have found that body-centered psychotherapy—a branch of psychotherapy that works from the premise that energy can be blocked or held in the body—is especially effective. The practitioners of body-centered psychotherapy have observed the connection between eye disorders and people's ability to express a variety of human emotions. They feel that the fixed stare that accompanies nearsightedness, for instance, can limit the range of sexual, visceral, and heart feelings that are communicated through the eyes.

Alexander Lowen, M.D., founder of bioenergetic therapy, states that patients suffering from myopia also have trouble making eye contact and expressing feelings through their eyes. Lowen believes that the emotional disturbance is primary to the vision impairment and the visual disturbance itself is secondary and a result of emotional strain.

Over time, this type of therapy often causes people's needed prescription for lenses to get lower and lower until they no longer need them. I have found the therapy is often quite helpful if used in conjunction with vision therapy, most especially in vision issues relating to abuse or abandonment.

Craniosacral Therapy

Craniosacral therapy is a hands-on system of treatment that uses palpation and gentle manipulation to evaluate a person's lack of flexibility and then restore flexibility to the central nervous system. Craniosacral therapy also treats connective tissue tension throughout the body, in order to restore the body to optimal tissue flexibility.

Osteopathic physicians, nurses, occupational and physical therapists, massage therapists, and other health care professionals may have training in craniosacral therapy.

Osteopaths and craniosacral therapists use their skills in palpation to detect problems, and their treatments can help patients improve their vision conditions. Strain patterns or imbalances of the craniosacral rhythm—also called the primary respiratory mechanism—can influence the eyes and have been found to be responsible for conditions including strabismus and refractive problems. These stresses respond beautifully to craniosacral therapy treatments.

Osteopathic treatments improve vision function as well as the physical health of the eye. Dr. W. G. Sutherland, founder of the practice of cranial osteopathy, and Dr. John Upledger have reported positive results for the treatment of various eye conditions, including strabismus, cataracts, and glaucoma. I have found these treatments to also be very successful for patients whose vision condition is rooted in head trauma.

Chiropractic Manipulation (Spinal Adjustments)

In my practice, I have found that people with vision problems greatly improve when spinal adjustments are added to vision therapy. Tension in the spinal cord, mechanical nerve pressure, and dislocated vertebrae can all be responsible for vision ailments, because they interfere with tissue nourishment and the nerve flow that the eyes need in order to function properly.

I find it to be especially important to pay attention to the upper cervical and midthoracic vertebrae, which supply the eyes with the nerve flow that is essential to vision. Chiropractic therapy too can be helpful in improving virtually all vision conditions.

Physical Exercise

Aerobic exercise not only benefits your heart, but it is also good for your eyes. Exercise raises the oxygen level in your cells and increases both lymph and blood circulation. As the body is made healthier in general, the eyes become healthier as well.

In my practice I use physical exercise as an adjunct to vision therapy. I recommend that you gently build up to aerobic exercise for a minimum of twenty minutes a day, four days a week. You don't have to join a health club, run five miles a day, or lift three hundred pounds in order to have good vision, but you do have to be active.

Here's what I recommend: Walk or jog. Get a good, comfortable pair of walking or running shoes and if possible, select a route that will not have you constantly pounding on concrete. Or, gently jump up and down every day on a minitrampoline. It keeps the blood flowing and improves circulation, especially in the legs and the head.

Physical exercise plays an important part in all my vision therapy programs. The type of exercise that I recommend depends upon the specific patient, his physical condition, and the nature of his vision situation.

Acupuncture

Acupuncture, a form of energy medicine, is the ancient Chinese medical practice of inserting needles into the skin at certain points of the body to improve, rebalance, or redirect the *qi* (also called *chi*), the life energy. Although the practice is more than five thousand years old, recent medical studies have proven its effectiveness.

How does it work? Chinese physicians conceived of specific points on the body as power points, junctures of pathways, called *meridians* that carry the human energy—the *qi*—throughout the body. These junctures are spots that are particularly sensitive to bioelectric impulses. When pressure (from the sister art of acupressure) or needles are applied to these points, energy blocks break down, energy is readily conducted throughout the body, and health is restored.

I have found acupuncture to help with all forms of vision disorders and to be of special help to my patients who are undergoing vision therapy.

Homeopathy

Another form of energy medicine that benefits patients suffering from any form of vision disorder is homeopathy.

A holistic medical science and healing art developed two hundred years ago by a German physician named Samuel Hahnemann, homeopathy is based on the principle that like cures like and employs the use of minute doses of natural remedies that are created from herbal, mineral, and animal substances.

It was Hahnemann's belief that symptoms of illness should never be suppressed, because they represent the body's efforts to repel and release disease. Just as mental health professionals have learned that the repression of emotion leads to illness, homeopathic practitioners have learned that the suppression of physical ailments leads to deeper and more serious disease conditions. Just as the suppression of symptoms leads to illness, the rapid and gentle expression of the same symptoms leads to cure.

While the techniques that are called homeopathic can be easily traced back to Hahnemann, the underlying principles of homeopathy can be traced back much further. It was Hippocrates himself, the Father of Medicine, who was the first to say that there were two methods of treating disease and that these two methods flowed as two healing streams, side by side but in opposite directions. The techniques used in both these healing streams are determined by the approach to and treatment of symptoms. Where allopathic medicine is largely concerned with the removal of pain and the treatment of the specific site of that pain, homeopathic healing is concerned with the treatment of the person experiencing pain and not with the treatment of the pain itself.

Therefore, while the allopath treats the disease, finding a medicine whose actions are in opposition to the patient's symptoms, the homeopath treats not the disease but the person. Where the allopath suppresses the symptoms of discomfort with the hope that the patient's vital force will ultimately heal his body, the homeopath treats by giving a remedy that would, in a healthy person, create the very symptoms that the patient is already experiencing. It is the homeopath's belief that as the patient's vital force rises up against the action of the remedy, not only will it move the patient to health, but it will also strengthen the patient's overall immunity against disease in general. This principle is called the Law of Similars and is stated as "Like cures like." It is the heart of homeopathic philosophy.

In practicing as they do, homeopaths work with a universal principle, one that we all learned in junior high school: for every action there is an equal and opposite reaction. In other words, any medicine will create a reaction within the human system, and the direction of overall weakness or strength is determined by the nature of that reaction.

Herbal Medicine

Long before there were drug companies and pharmacies, people grew herbs for medicinal purposes. Modern researchers are now confirming that herbs have an enormous and exciting range of healing powers and that they can be a safe, natural, and inexpensive alternative to synthetic drugs. Plus, when properly prescribed they have few side effects.

Herbal medicine is another treatment modality that takes a holistic approach to healing, viewing the patient as a whole rather than as an accumulation of body parts.

When appropriate, I have referred patients to a qualified herbalist as a part of vision treatment.

The Alexander Technique

Frederick Matthias Alexander was one of the first people to notice how faulty posture—including sitting, moving, and standing—is connected with serious physical and emotional problems. Pioneering a simple, effective approach to rebalancing the body through awareness, movement, and touch, he was aware that the correct relationship of the head, neck, and back is essential for proper movement and functioning. Alexander observed that people habitually "misuse" their bodies, and he developed a system to help them become conscious of their faulty habits. His patients learned how to interrupt or inhibit familiar postural "sets" that correspond to these habits so that their bodies could be guided to improved motion and balance.

In my practice, I have found that the rebalancing process can be very helpful to vision health.

Feldenkrais Method

Moshe Feldenkrais was a physicist who did nuclear radiation research in France and England. He is best known, though, in the field of bodywork. Feldenkrais coined the term self-image and believed that each of us speaks, moves, thinks, and feels in a unique way, according to the image that we hold of ourselves. In order to change our mode of action, we must first change that image that binds us to past behaviors, including illness.

Feldenkrais viewed the human organism as a complex system of intelligence and function, in which all movement reflects the state of the nervous system. This is also the basis of self-awareness. You become accustomed to your movements, whether they are good or bad, and this can lead to a number of physical and emotional problems. He reasoned that if the negative habitual patterns of movement are interrupted, the body will learn to function at greater ease and fluidity. This, in turn, improves your self-image and increases awareness and health.

He recognized the importance of breath and viewed it as an integral form of movement. Poor movement and poor functioning impair the breathing, and improper breathing interferes with the proper functioning of the body. He found that even the movement of the eyes could seriously interfere with how the other parts of the body function.

By increasing your awareness of how you move and by helping free the eyes of any contractions in their movement, the Feldenkrais method is a helpful adjunct to a vision therapy protocol.

Therapeutic Massage

Muscle tension, from normal activity, awkward movement, or stress, contributes to muscle fatigue and pain by compressing nerve fibers in the muscle. Prolonged contraction interferes with the elimination of chemical wastes in the muscles and surrounding tissues and can cause frequent nerve and muscle pain. If not properly addressed, these body tensions have a tendency to build into chronic patterns of stress.

Prolonged tension can cause pain in other parts of the body. Headaches, for instance, often are caused by overly tense muscles of the neck, shoulders, and lower back. Massage can break up these muscular waste deposits and stimulate circulation.

I have found massage to be an excellent general adjunct for the patients who come to me for natural vision improvement.

Rolfing

The Rolfing technique is based on the concept that all human function improves when the segments of the body—the head, the torso, the pelvis, the legs, and the feet—are properly aligned. This state of balance and alignment is called structural integration. Biochemist Ida Rolf, Ph.D., the developer of the technique, believed that balance could be reestablished by the manual manipulation—specifically, the stretching—of the body's fascial tissues. The *fascia* is a thin, elastic, semifluid membrane and envelops every muscle, bone, nerve, blood vessel, and organ. It plays an integral role in maintaining posture and proper movement.

I have found Rolfing to be helpful to patients whose bodies hold a great deal of tension. But note that this is a very deep form of bodywork and not for everyone.

Yoga

The term *yoga* literally means "union." It is so named because its practice leads to the integration of the physical, mental, and spiritual energies that together enhance health and well-being. Yoga teaches the basic principle of mind-body unity. If the mind is chronically restless and agitated, the health of the body will be compromised, and if the body is in poor health, mental clarity and strength will be adversely affected. The practice of yoga can counter these ill effects, restoring mental and physical health.

I don't know anyone who would not benefit from the discipline of yoga. I recommend it often to my patients.

Meditation

I define meditation as "any activity that keeps your attention in the present moment." When your mind is calm and focused in the present, it is neither reacting to memories of the past nor preoccupied with plans for the future. The simplest form of meditation is to sit quietly and focus your attention on the rhythm of your own breath. The connection between your breath and your state of mind is a basic principle of both yoga and meditation. When you are anxious, frightened, or agitated, your breath tends to become more rapid, shallow, and uneven. On the other hand, when your mind is calm and focused, your breathing will tend to be slower, deeper, and more regular. Focusing your mind on your inhalation and exhalation provides a natural rhythm for meditation and for keeping in the present moment. As a result, your mind will become both more tranquil and more aware.

As with yoga, I believe that everyone both responds to and benefits from meditation.

Nutrition

Finally, there is nutrition. We have all heard that eating carrots is good for our eyes. Although that is true, it is just a part of what good nutrition can mean to you and your eyes.

Consider this fact: more than 25 percent of the nutrients that you absorb from your food go to nourishing your visual system—the eyes plus the nerves, blood vessels, and tissues that support vision. Therefore, proper nutrition may be of greater importance to your eyes than it is to any other part of your body.

What do I mean by good nutrition? First and foremost, I mean balance—it is essential that you eat a balanced variety of whole foods. Your body does not use individual vitamins and minerals in isolation. They are absorbed and used in clusters. Therefore, the absence of one nutrient can affect your body's ability to use another.

Yet, today, it is probably not realistic to expect to get all of your nutrients from food alone. No matter how wholesome and pure your food might be, there are factors that affect its full content—how it is grown, how it is stored, and how it is cooked, among others. Besides, science determines the value under ideal laboratory conditions. What your body actually absorbs can be very different. Your age, health, activity level, and stress can all affect both what your body needs and how well it can take what it needs from your diet.

Therefore, in addition to carefully monitoring what you eat, I recommend that you take vitamin and mineral supplements in order to enhance your vision.

A Case of Mixed Modalities

Paul, a forty-year-old stockbroker, was an important, busy man, who was constantly on the go. Whether working, playing sports, or partying, he gave it 110 percent. His primary reason for coming into my office was that his nearsightedness was getting a little worse and his eyes hurt after he spent a few hours on his computer.

The recent increase in Paul's nearsightedness and his eyestrain were both a reflection of how he operated in life. I recommended vision therapy, conventional corrective lenses, and other modalities of treatment. I told him that we could not successfully treat just his eyes; we had to treat the person behind the eyes as well.

When I tried to discuss nutrition with Paul, he told me that he ate a good deal of fast food and that his car was his primary dining room. After years of eating doughnuts and coffee while sitting in a traffic jam, he had recently begun to have trouble with his digestion as well.

When we discussed exercise, Paul told me that he loved playing sports and always looked forward to his twice-weekly basketball games at the gym and that he tried to exercise every day but sometimes did not have the time.

When I put together Paul's personal vision care program, I recommended the following: In order to take the strain off Paul's eyes while he sat in front of the computer, I recommended a pair of computer glasses, separate from his distance vision glasses or contact lenses. These glasses took the pressure off his eye muscles while he was doing any close work, including reading.

Paul's vision therapy program was designed to help him develop more flexibility in his focusing and eye-teaming skills. The core of the program centered on Paul's learning to relax not only his eyes but his mind and body as well. I gave him a series of exercises, some of which were to be performed daily and others only once or twice a week. I told him to approach the exercises not as a form of physical exercise like weight training but in the manner of meditation.

As for his lifestyle, I told Paul that he had to cut down or, best, eliminate alcohol, coffee, and the occasional cigar. He had to cut back on fast food, pastries, fried foods, and high-fat meals. I recommended that he eat more fruits, vegetables, and, as a snack, whole-grain energy bars. I stressed that he make time daily to sit and eat quietly and that he eat more slowly in order to take the stress off his digestive system.

For an exercise program, I suggested that Paul get a minimum of twenty minutes of some type of aerobic exercise daily, like running or using an exercise bike or StairMaster, in order to give him an outlet for his pent-up energy.

I also suggested strongly that Paul try to meditate, even for only five minutes a day. He reported back to me later that this was the hardest part of his treatment, as he attempted to be and not do. Paul's favorite of my recommendations was that he have a massage at least once a week. Once he tried it, he was hooked. He had deep-tissue massage, or shiatsu, weekly.

In following this integrated approach to his vision problems, Paul soon discovered that he was able to reduce the prescription required for his nearsightedness and to all but eliminate the stress in his life. In addition, Paul's digestive disorders soon disappeared, and he reported that he was feeling better as a person.

CHAPTER 7

Defining
Greater Vision

The Philosophy of Natural Vision Improvement

"Here lies Salvino degli Armati, Inventor of Spectacles.
May God pardon him for his sins."

—Inscribed on a tomb in the
church of Santa Maria
Maggiore, Florence, Italy

istory cannot clearly show whether or not the Florentines
were correct in their belief that Salvino degli Armati indeed
was the inventor of glasses. But there is a good bit of proof
that they were quite correct in damning him for his actions.

Over the centuries, there has been much discussion as to who was
the first person to make a pair of glasses. We know that the Egyptians
busied themselves with vision therapy. They corrected eye-teaming
problems with the use of a mask that had two small eyeholes in it placed
far apart. The idea was that the overconvergent patient would have to
work hard to have his two eyes see out of the holes.

The idea of vision therapy, in fact, predates the concept of glasses
by thousands of years. Many of us live with the misconception that
vision therapy—or, to name it more correctly, natural vision improve-

ment—was invented at the beginning of the last century by a man named William Bates. But while Bates certainly had a huge impact upon the idea that we could learn to see better naturally if we would only exercise both our eyes and our vision, he was certainly not the creator of the concept.

The concept of vision therapy, of improving how we perceive the world visually, was perhaps the work of Greek philosophers, who were themselves trying to understand the world.

They understood vision to be a dynamic process, one that involves an interaction, a relationship, between the viewer and the viewed. Plato himself insisted that the eyes not only took in energy but sent it forth as well. And he insisted that the visual system not only took in images but perceived information as well. Plato believed that the aspect of self that actually perceived the world was the human soul.

By the time of the Roman Empire, the concept of naturally improving vision had, to some degree, been replaced through the use of corrective lenses. It is doubtful that actual pairs of glasses were being made, but Pliny reports that Nero used a concave gem set in a ring that he placed before his eye in order to see the games in the Coliseum in Rome.

Shaping the History of Natural Vision Improvement

Why the controversy about glasses? As William Bates himself wrote in his book *Perfect Sight Without Glasses*, "If, however, his contemporaries believed that Salvino of the Armati was the first to produce these aids to vision, they might well pray for the pardon of his sins; for while it is true that eyeglasses have brought to some people improved vision and relief from pain and discomfort, they have been to others simply an added torture. They always do more or less harm, and at their best they never improve vision to normal."

That last is the key. In today's world, the eye care profession tends to take vision problems in stride. In fact, many eye doctors focus their attention so much on accommodation and the clarity of the image itself that they tend not to even diagnose many other forms of vision disorder, such as eye teaming or suppression of the image in an eye. Instead, they slap a pair of glasses on their patients' faces.

Don't get me wrong. Unlike the citizens of ancient Florence, I don't think glasses are always an evil thing. But I am aware, and I want you to be aware as well, that a pair of glasses never fixed the vision problems of a pair of eyes—quite the opposite. Because that pair of lenses makes everything clear and makes better vision possible, the eyes behind the lenses actually stop trying so hard to see. They let the lenses do the seeing for them. That is why, a year or so later, you might need another pair of glasses with stronger lenses.

When considering the workings of the world, it is important to remember that the Greek philosophers did not say to themselves, "What can be put in front of the eyes in order to make vision clearer?" They instead asked, "How can we help these eyes to see more clearly, to perceive more correctly?"

George Berkley, in his eighteenth-century "Essay Toward a New Theory of Vision," insisted upon a philosophy that vision was more than just an optical event. He wrote that the ability to perceive distance was not something that happened in the eye alone, but that it needed to be integrated between the eye and the brain.

Berkley was lauded for his work with the blind. He wrote, "When a congenitally blind person was surgically given sight, he was, at first, so far from making any judgment about distances that he thought all objects touched his eyes. . . . He knew not the shape of anything, nor any one thing from another, however different in shape or magnitude." This observation gave rise to the idea that the judgment of distance is something more than an innate ability.

During this same time period, the philosopher Spinoza gave additional insight into how vision really works. He theorized that the image the eyes see is affected by past experience and therefore affected both by memory (the interpretation of past experience) and by beliefs (or biases). Spinoza also theorized that mind and body could not be separated, since they were one and the same.

The idea of natural vision improvement was further refined in the teachings of modern-era philosophers George Gurdjieff and his student Ouspensky. Each spoke a good deal on the subject of self-observation, a concept that posits "to know others, one must first know oneself." Thus, self-observation is the key to awareness and attention.

Both go on to state that to really know yourself properly, "one must first of all remember oneself." This remembering is a nonanalytical way of directing attention onto yourself without weakening or detracting your attention from other things.

Ouspensky illustrates his point using an arrow that extends from you and points to what you observe:

I $\longrightarrow$ the observed phenomenon

If, however, while observing, you try to remember yourself, you direct attention toward both the object and yourself. He illustrates this point by using a line with two arrows that connect you with what you observe:

I $\longleftrightarrow$ the observed phenomenon

Understanding that there will be a great resistance to remembering yourself, Ouspensky advises that the first step you should take is to realize that you are fully conscious all the time. "When we realize this and observe it for some time, we must try to catch ourselves at the moments when we are not conscious, and little by little, this will make us more conscious."

In other words, by suggesting that you observe yourself as you are in the process of observing and perceiving the world around you, Gurdjieff and Ouspensky are advising that you live in the present moment. This, of course, is part of the philosophy of natural vision improvement and an important part in attaining greater vision.

Krishnamurti said, "You must begin to observe and listen, not only to what is being said but also to your distortions. As you are observing, see your prejudices, your opinions, your images, your experiences, and see how they prevent you from observing."

Carlos Casteneda wrote that by "talking to ourselves too much and by repeating the same talk and the same choices over and over again, we maintain our world." For Casteneda, a warrior is the person of knowledge, the person who knows the effects of this inner dialogue and seeks to end the inner chatter. A warrior "listens to the world . . . and . . . is aware that the world will change as soon as he stops talking to himself." In terms of greater vision, your internal chatter lessens as you are more in your own vision and less inside your own head.

The philosophy of traditional Chinese medicine provides another important tool in shaping my practice of natural vision improvement. Traditional Chinese medicine is based in the wonderful concept that you cannot measure static things in order to find answers for your problems and to understand the root cause of a problem you need to look at interactions and relationships. Chinese doctors look for patterns of disharmony. For them, direct cause and effect is secondary to the overall pattern of nature. Traditional Chinese doctors don't ask "How does X cause Y?" Instead they ask, "What is the relationship between X and Y?"

The Chinese model is a holistic one, based on the idea that no single part can be understood except in relation to the whole. A symptom is not traced back to the cause but is looked upon as a part of the totality.

Again, this beautifully informs the concept of greater vision, a concept that will apply all of the above to the practice of natural vision improvement.

The History of Vision Training

As has been previously stated, the art of vision training dates back to early man, most likely to the ancient Greeks or Egyptians. But the first doctor to step forth and announce that vision could and should be perfected naturally, through exercise and not through the use of glasses, was William H. Bates, M.D.

William Bates

William Bates was a respected New York ophthalmologist who lived from 1860 to 1931. He was a graduate of the College of Physicians and Surgeons at Columbia University. And from 1886 to 1891, he was an instructor of ophthalmology at the New York Postgraduate Medical School and Hospital.

From 1919 until 1930, he published a monthly magazine called *Better Eyesight*. In 1920, he published his book, *Perfect Sight Without Glasses*. He was the founder of the Bates system, a method of training by which specific eye exercises were used to improve vision. Bates not only was an eye doctor; he was also a scientist of some import. And he approached his work in vision training from a scientific standpoint. He investigated why vision changed for the worse by examining patients in many different emotional states. And he noted how emotions seemed to have a direct impact upon vision. He wrote of many cases in which patients' nearsightedness or farsightedness would change as their mood changed.

He concluded ultimately that the eyeball itself must be able to change shape, though this was a hard conclusion for him to make, because it disputed everything that he had learned in medical school.

Writing in the April 1923 issue of *Better Eyesight*, L. L. Biddle gives some background of Bates's early work:

> For the benefit of those who were unable to attend Dr. Bates' lecture before the New York Association of Osteopaths at the Wal-

dorf Astoria on Saturday evening, February 17, I decided to take down a few notes which I will now try to compile.

The chairman introduced Dr. Bates by stating that the osteopaths take away the crutches, and Dr. Bates takes away the glasses. . . .

He [Bates] then commenced by telling how he made his first discoveries and cited the opposition he had to buck against. He stated that his attitude of mind, ever since he was a little boy, was to find out all the facts possible about a subject and then to work on these as a basis, rather than on a guess or theory. When he commenced practicing medicine in 1885, one of his first patients who came to him had a slight degree of myopia or nearsightedness. Upon examining his eyes, he found that the patient was not nearsighted all of the time. When the patient would look at a blank wall and not try to see anything, his eyes for short periods were normal. He persuaded this patient to go without his glasses, and his eyes reached a point where they stayed normal all of the time.

Dr. Bates said that he then started boasting around the hospital about the improvement. However, it got so on the house surgeon's nerves that he brought up a ward patient who was nearsighted, and with that patient, Bates managed equal success. Much to his surprise, instead of the doctors praising him and trying to find out how he accomplished these heretofore impossible improvements, Dr. Bates suddenly became very unpopular with the rest of the staff. These successes nevertheless spurred him on in his experiments at the New York Aquarium and at the laboratory of the Columbia College of Physicians and Surgeons, and as a result, he discovered that the accommodation of the eye is not brought about by a change in the shape of the lens, but by the lengthening and shortening of the eyeball itself, as the bellows of a camera.

Due to his theories, Bates was expelled from the University. This was quite a handicap, but he obtained a small laboratory for himself and continued his work.

Controversial to the end, Bates insisted that his experiments proved that patients' prescriptions were not fixed but could and did change depending upon their emotional states. And even though he would document case after case for years, he was never able to get the medical community at large to accept his theories.

The Bates method presents the patient with a series of exercises that were designed to be of no harm to anyone who did them. Bates's intent in the design of his system was to create a number of exercises that were for the general good of the public. He felt that a person with any eye condition could do his exercises, possibly with vision improvement and certainly with no harm. While all the exercises could be done by all people, some of them were geared to specific disorders.

The Bates method proved to be very popular because it presented the possibility of patients seeing clearly without glasses. Note that at the early part of the last century, glasses were not popular fashion accessories like they are now. With their plastic frames and glass lenses, they were both heavy and unattractive. Those wearing them were commonly called "four eyes," and young women of the day were reminded that "men seldom make passes at girls who wear glasses." So the enticement of being able to toss away those glasses and see clearly was potent indeed.

One of the most famous advocates of the Bates method was Aldous Huxley, the British novelist who, while working with Bates's student Margaret Corbett, wrote a book titled *The Art of Seeing* about his own experience with natural vision improvement.

Among the core questions raised by Bates about traditional eye care had to do with glasses. Why, Bates asked, if prescription lenses corrected vision defects, did a patient ever need stronger glasses?

Bates concluded that glasses only artificially correct vision defects and in doing so actually contribute to the deterioration of vision and of the eyes. In his book *Better Eyesight Without Glasses* he wrote, "Corrective lenses require the eye to strain to the exact prescription level in order to see correctly. . . . The precise center of the lens is the place of best sight and therefore causes the wearer to hold the eyes rather fixed and immobile looking through the center, turning the head rather than the eyes." He felt that this accounted for the "stuck look" in the eyes of many nearsighted people who wear corrective lenses full-time.

Bates's theory was that tension in the extraocular muscles of the eyes was responsible for difficulties with sight. He felt that these muscles, which are responsible for moving the eye up and down and left and right, could either flatten or enlarge next to the eyeball, depending upon where the eyes were focused.

Bates thought, therefore, that the reason patients needed prescription glasses was that they misused the extraocular muscles and that the primary way to help with the tension caused by this misuse was to train the muscles to relax with a series of exercises. Once relaxed, the muscles would function correctly.

In his theory of eyesight, Bates also believed that the muscles surrounding the eye consisted of conscious muscles, which could be trained to act on direct command, and unconscious muscles, which could only imitate the actions of the conscious muscles. Thus, one of the goals of Bates's therapy was to train his patients in the control of the conscious muscles, believing that then the unconscious muscles would follow their lead. Note that Bates's theory, formed in the early part of the twentieth century, was confirmed in scientific fact in 1964.

Overall, Bates presented three principles for natural vision improvement. The first—aptly called movement—was that the eyes are made for movement and that all sense perception is based in movement. He found through his research that when we are placed under stress, our movement tends to slow to a stare. Our breathing rate also tends to slow as we intensify visual concentration.

Bates's second principle was called centralization. It states that the human mind and eyes together develop a skill for directing their full attention at one specific, central point at a time, since the human eye can see only one point clearly at a time.

And his third principle was called relaxation. Bates felt that vision, as a process, is 90 percent mental and 10 percent physical. He felt that if patients have to strain to see, they will cause tension in their entire visual system. Bates said, "You can teach people how to produce any error in refraction, how to produce a crossed eye, how to see two images of an object . . . at any angle from each other, simply by teaching them how to think in a particular way."

Bates believed that in order to improve vision, it was essential to develop the mind's ability to visualize. In fact, nearly all of the exercises in the Bates method integrate movement, breathing, awareness, and relaxation with imagery.

Bates stressed the importance of patients' being conscious of their breathing when doing his eye exercises, or at least being aware of when they begin to hold their breath. He also spoke of the importance of blinking, not only to lubricate the eyeballs but also to prevent the tendency to stare while performing a visual task.

That Bates's method was based on an interrelationship of movement, awareness, relaxation, and visualization as they affect visual function and human behavior makes him one of the pioneers in the history of natural vision improvement. His work has greatly informed the philosophy and practice of greater vision.

A. M. Skeffington

Just a few years after the Bates method began to gain popularity, the field of behavioral optometry was founded by A. M. Skeffington, O.D. A graduate of the Needles Institute of Optometry in Kansas City, Missouri, in 1917, Skeffington had been trained within the same medical model as Bates, and like Bates, he came to challenge that model. Skeffington believed that the behavior of individuals had to be taken into account when prescribing them glasses. In 1928, he became the educational director for the Optometric Extension Program (OEP), which developed a curriculum for training students of behavioral optometry. Today, the OEP is an internationally recognized organization that informs both professionals and the public about the importance of vision in their lives.

In the 1930s, Skeffington met a research scientist named Emmett Betts. Together they developed a program that enlarged the role of the optometrist to include early learning work, specifically in helping children to read better. This groundbreaking work continues today.

Throughout the thirties and forties, Skeffington continued to develop the field of behavioral optometry, incorporating into the field the study of the psychological aspects of vision and the role of body posture in vision distortions.

To his dying day, Skeffington continued to develop the field of behavioral optometry. Among the most important principles of the field are as follows:

1. Take time with people: Skeffington taught that each individual is unique. In order to gain a full understanding of how individuals' visual systems relate to their needs, an optometrist must spend a sufficient amount of time with them.
2. Be humanistic: Skeffington taught that it was essential that an optometrist genuinely care for people. The optometrist who delivers vision care without emotion delivers vision care that is empty, pointless. The optometrist must empathize with the patients' difficulties and struggles.
3. Be therapeutic: He also taught that treatment procedures must outweigh diagnostic procedures. The very heart of optometry is to provide improvement of visual functioning. It follows that emphasis be placed on accomplishing visual improvement. A diagnosis is not an end in itself; it is a means toward the more primary goal of treatment.
4. Be contemporary: Skeffington taught that knowledge does not stand still. Maintaining knowledge requires a peripheral awareness of new trends, new ideas, and new ways of thinking. Optometrists must be continually sensitive to contemporary issues. They must evaluate older ideas in the realm of current thought. If necessary, they must discard older ideas in the light of new knowledge.
5. Be controversial: Skeffington believed that a profession cannot be at the cutting edge of new developments in medical care without being willing to accept the inherent controversy that comes with this stance.

6. Be holistic: Skeffington taught that vision does not exist in isolation from the rest of the body or, indeed, from the world. This requires optometry to be aware of related areas that impact visual function. The blending of knowledge from other professions with the optometrists' own enables the care they render to be more thorough and effective.

7. Be creative: Skeffington taught that no two patients have exactly the same needs. Therefore, no two patients are to be treated in exactly the same way. Optometrists must be creative in their approaches so that they may tap into the individual nature of their patients. They must get at what allows patients to move ahead and improve their visual function.

8. Recognize your impact: Finally, Skeffington taught that society places a high premium on visual performance and that vision permeates an incredibly large number of activities in daily life. Therefore, Skeffington wanted optometrists to always be aware of the importance of their work and the need for their work to be as excellent as it could be. As his own wife said about him, Skeffington admonished his students to "accomplish all they felt needed to get done."

Emile Javal

It wasn't until the late 1800s that orthoptics was created. *Orthoptics*, which literally means "straight eyes," was a discipline created specifically for eye-teaming issues—to help the two eyes to work together. French ophthalmologist Emile Javal was responsible for laying the foundation for modern orthoptics.

Javal was motivated to begin his work when his sister and father each had eye surgery—the results of which he described as *le massacre des muscles oculaires*, or the massacre of his family's eyes. Javal designed procedures to treat binocular problems without surgery.

Even today, with all our modern technology, the success rate for binocularity issues is about 70 percent with vision therapy. This is, of course, opposed to the 20 percent success rate of surgery.

Orthoptics is based upon the principle that the eye muscles can be reprogrammed through the use of eye exercises. But since the eye and brain are so integrated in their functioning, it is really the eye-brain connection and not the eye itself that is trained in exercises.

During the 1920s, optometric visual training began to be practiced, with the concepts of orthoptics as its basis. Visual training was defined as "the art and science of developing visual skills to achieve optimal visual performance and comfort." Even people without turned eyes were doing eye exercises in an effort to maximize their vision. The treatment can be as simple as patching an eye, or it can involve the use of equipment ranging from old-fashioned stereoscopes—devices that allow people to see three-dimensionally in an artificial environment—to modern computers. It is done today as it has always been done, both in the home and the doctor's office.

Today, vision training combines the work in visual clarity developed by Bates with Javal's program to develop eye teaming. Along the way, it has come to include the vision therapy developed by the U.S. military during World War II to improve soldiers' ability to target and to make split-second decisions. And new tools—like the Accommotrac discussed in Chapter 6—have developed, and new methods of treatment have been found.

Note that the practice of vision therapy tends to vary greatly from office to office.

In the pages of the next chapter, I will share how my own philosophy of vision therapy has changed over the years and how I practice it now.

CHAPTER 8

Attaining Greater Vision

The Practice of Natural Vision Improvement

"When we see through authentically powered eyes, metaphorically speaking, one has more ability to see without obstruction, more ability to live love and wisdom, and more ability and desire to help others evolve into the same love and light."

—Gary Zukav, *The Seat of the Soul*

In my office, I practice a form of medicine combining behavioral optometry, vision therapy, and traditional Chinese medicine that offers my patients a unique take on vision care. My over twenty years' clinical experience has also informed my own unique style of natural vision improvement. I believe in combining early vision tools such as the stereoscope and the simple eye patch with cutting-edge computerized machinery in order to offer my patients a system of vision therapy that is at once challenging, supportive, and dynamic.

When you sit in my waiting room, you are likely to hear laughter from one room, sobs from another, and the dead silence of concentration from a third. I find it of vital importance that my office be a workplace that is also a *safe* place, a place in which the patient who is uncovering the core issues of his vision disorder is free to feel whatever he feels and to express it openly. Thus, boxes of Kleenex abound, as does a sense of discovery and growth.

As I often work with young children with learning disabilities, the waiting room floor is likely to be littered with multicolored blocks that have been assembled into free-form coliseums hither and yon.

Overall, it seems a place of ever-so-slightly controlled chaos. And it is just as it should be.

Getting to Shen

When a patient first comes to my office, I look her straight in the eyes, not only in order to begin gathering information on her condition but also to establish contact, to begin building a bridge of trust between us.

I begin scanning for information, and I notice the energy in her eyes. Is it alive and powerful, or is it remote, dull? I seek to understand what percentage of her own vital force, or *qi*, she makes available to herself and what percentage she sends out into the world.

As I look at each eye, I ask myself whether this eye wants to participate in life or to retreat. Often, I notice that one eye is powerful and outgoing, while the other seems to be listless and remote.

I can remember once saying to a patient that her left eye was like an old woman's; it was still alive, but it was tired and withdrawn and didn't want to participate in life anymore.

I've seen eyes that seemed to be frozen in a constant state of shock. This sometimes happens after patients have been through a traumatic event. Their eyes will literally seem to have frozen at the instant of a car accident. Their bodies may have recuperated and may be active and alive in the present moment, but the images taken in through their eyes are still frozen in their unconscious mind, as well as in the physical structure of the eyes.

Such an event can cause these patients to have a constant, unconscious sense of anxiety that they carry with them like a fifty-pound weight. I call this syndrome eyeballs trapped in time. I use this term because I have found that during a traumatic event, the eyes watch together in fear of the oncoming tragedy. It may be a traffic accident involving a head-on collision, an object falling from above to the right or left, or any other trauma. When the eyes witness the oncoming trauma, they record and hold the image of the event, and the patients' awareness of time shifts—time seems to slow down. Sometimes the time shift happens to both eyes equally; sometimes it affects one eye more than the other. From that moment, the change of time sense can be locked into that eye or to both eyes. Left untreated, this sense of frozen time can inhibit the patients' vision from that day forward.

Just as physical trauma can leave its mark on patients' eyes, so can emotional trauma. The death of a loved one, the end of a love relationship, the loss of a career, or moving from one home to another are all events that can create enough emotional impact to affect patients' vision and leave their mark on their eyes as well.

After I get a sense of my patient's state of being, I use this information to select the eye tests that will best provide insight into his vision disorder and how to go about correcting it. These tests will also help me determine how I can set up the all-important safe place in which that patient can work his way back to health.

Remember, every person who comes into the office is, for me, a new adventure, since everyone's vision is their own unique representation of a life's path. Each patient has his or her own distinctive way of thinking, feeling, being, and seeing in the world. Each set of eyes perceives a different world from mine. Their past, present, and dreams for the future all greatly determine how they see and "be" in the world.

What makes my patients' vision unique to them? My own study of Chinese medicine, homeopathy, and other forms of medicine that involve character typing have led me to believe that at the core level, they came into the world attached to certain basic energies that flow through them.

The flow of these basic energies in each of their unique systems influences how they live their lives, what kind of relationships they have, what kind of career paths they follow, what fears they have, what their life's desires are, and so much more of their life experiences. I believe that each patient's flow of energy is his or hers uniquely. They were born with it, and their vision will be shaped by it. In my practice I work with these basic energies, healing my patients' physical sense of sight by first healing their spiritual sense of vision. I call this process "getting to shen," *shen* being the word in traditional Chinese medicine for "spirit."

The practice of greater vision—the process of attaining unlimited freedom of clarity and comprehension—gives patients a deeper understanding of how their own vision is a tool and how they can use it to begin an adventure and live their life without limits. They come to understand how they have seen the world and how their worldview has shaped their personal reality. I explain to them that vision is really just about seeing and being in a relationship with themselves and with their world.

By developing this expanded sense of vision, my patients are able to accept more responsibility for their lives, instead of being swept away by the energies of the people around them. They discover that the state of greater vision depends upon living in harmony within the world.

Most importantly, they learn to know themselves. Many of the deepest vision problems come from stress upon the physical, emotional, and spiritual levels of our lives, from living in a way that people know is in conflict with their true natures.

As the *I Ching* says, "If the individual acts consistently and is true to himself, he will find the way that is appropriate for him. . . . This is right for him and without blame." This is what I have always loved about the *I Ching* and what I have tried to carry over to my program of vision therapy: no blame.

Testing Eyes, Testing Vision

The following are some of the tests that I do in order to evaluate a patient's vision.

The Cover Test

This is a very quick and simple test that can reveal a great deal. I hold a pencil tip approximately sixteen inches away from the patient's face on the midline of her nose. I ask her to look at the pencil tip, and I notice whether she looks hard at the pencil or holds it easily with her eyes. I notice if it is easy for her to target the pencil or hard for her to move her eyes onto the target. I watch the split-second process by which she moves her eyes, locks on target, and then holds the target. It tells me a great deal about the person and her eyes.

Then I take a small paddle and alternately cover and then uncover each eye, while the patient is still targeting the pencil. As I move the paddle from eye to eye, I notice how the eye that has been covered moves when it is again uncovered. Has it remained steady and on target, or has it wandered about while covered?

I ask the patient if when the eye was uncovered, it seemed to her that the pencil had moved or stayed still. I note whether or not she reports that the pencil moved in the same direction as the eye had moved. I also observe if the sensation of movement is merely horizontal or if it is also vertical.

The cover test allows me to observe what happens to the patient's eyes when they are each allowed to go into a rest position. Once I have covered an eye, it can no longer do its job—so what does it try to do? I call this rest position the soul position, because it reveals to me how the eye sees itself when it is not asked to perform any action. Does it quickly return to participate in life when the paddle is moved, or does it take its time, coming back in wary steps, not sure whether it can trust the world or not?

Then I ask myself, "Is there a difference in the way that the two eyes reacted?" If so, I record how great that difference was. If there is a marked difference between the actions of the two eyes and if there is also an observable difference in the spirit of the eyes, I consider the possibility that the patient may be exhibiting a split personality. I then check her pulse in the manner set forth in traditional Chinese medicine. This is to get a reading of the energies in the patient's various organ systems, which allows me to understand how united the aspects of that patient's life are within her being.

For example, I had a patient who showed a marked difference in the energies given off by each eye and how each eye reacted to the cover test. One eye came back on-line very quickly, returning to look at the target, while the other eye took a good deal of time.

I asked that patient if he ever felt like he had two different people living in the same body. He answered me with a sly smile, "Yes, of course." He continued by saying, "Many times during the day I feel I have one part that wants to nourish and another that wants to destroy me." He told me that it was his pattern that if he ate something he knew was good for his system, he would accompany it with a drink that he knew to be bad. In the same way, his entire life was a balancing act of nurturing and destructive acts.

If people are disintegrated, like that patient, they tend to experience life as a roller coaster of highs and lows, each peak and valley representing a part of their own nature. Once this has been diagnosed, it becomes the job of the vision therapist to help them to understand both aspects of their nature and to work to unify them.

Near Visual Space Test

For this little test, I hold the pencil tip about twenty inches from the patient's eyes, at a point even with his nose. I then ask the patient to look at the tip of the pencil, and I notice how easy it is for him to target that tip.

Then I begin to move the pencil slowly toward the patient's nose and ask him to tell me about anything he feels or sees while still targeting that now-moving tip.

I purposely keep my instructions vague and simple so that the patient can fill in whatever information he finds important. Often, it will give me an idea of what his personal awareness is like. He may say, "I see two pencils," or "This makes my eyes hurt." A look of strain may appear on his face, or his whole body might tense up and retreat from the pencil as it moves toward his eyes. He may be very sensitive to the test, or he may feel and notice nothing.

I repeat the test three times with both eyes together, then three times with each eye separately.

When the test is performed with both eyes, it is especially important that I learn whether or not the patient saw a double image. This doubling means that one of the eyes has diverged from the target. At the point at which the image becomes double, I stop moving forward and move the target swiftly back toward me until the patient says that he sees the target singly.

The test shows how well the patient can cope with the world coming at him, as well as how well he can cope with the sensation of speed. There is, metaphorically, a whole world in that pencil tip. When it moves swiftly toward him, he shows how well he adapts to the world's intrusions. Does he break down, as with the double image? Does he strive and strive, in an effort to stay in contact with the world? Does he react in any number of other ways: with pain (headache), with fear, with anger, with numbness, or with some other emotion?

This test also gives an indication as to the size and shape of the patient's personal space. At what point does the patient begin to react to the moving target? How does the motion affect his breathing? How does it impact upon the tension in his body?

This exercise can also indicate the balance between the two eyes. How do the eyes react individually to the motion of the target? Is there a big difference between the reactions of each eye to the test?

Finally, I purposely repeat this test three times to see the patient's ability to maintain concentration. If the patient's attention erodes each time I perform the test, his visual system is easily exhausted by doing any sort of task, like reading.

Repetition also shows how the patient may compensate for a weakened visual system. Often, the patient who does worse on the second testing will bounce back for the third. On some level, the patient is aware of the weakness and works to overcome it with increased concentration. This type of patient most often is strong-willed and a quick learner.

Overall, this test gives me insight into how the individual is able to make contact with the world and how easily he lets other individuals into his personal space. It also defines the individual's sensory boundaries and how strong-willed he is.

The Eye Chart Test

As in every other office, in my office the eye chart is the standard twenty feet away from the patient. I ask the patient to read the chart without glasses or contact lenses. While she reads, I notice whether she is straining or looking easily at the chart, as well as how effectively she is targeting the chart as a whole and the individual letters on the chart.

I have the patient read with both eyes together and with each eye individually. Then I repeat the test, having the patient use her glasses and/or contact lenses.

Again, as we begin, I'm purposely vague in my instructions. I only ask the patient to read the chart. I notice where she chooses to begin—larger letters or smaller letters. I notice if she skips letters. I notice the smallest letters that she is able to read with and without her glasses.

This test reveals how well a patient is able to direct her looking—the ability to target with the eyes. It also reflects the patient's skill at seeing—the ability to identify the target with her mind. It ultimately reveals how much space the patient can deal with at any one time and still be able to understand what is being taken in.

It is also, of course, an exercise in clarity and reveals how clearly she is able to see in the twenty feet, which is the usual size of a human's sensory awareness boundary.

Eye Movement Tests

In any vision exam, it is essential that the practitioner assess how well the patient can move his eyes to scan the environment and to follow moving targets.

To test saccadic eye movements, I have the patient stand or sit directly in front of me. I hold two small targets, one black and one white, about sixteen inches in front of the patient's face. Each target is about four inches to the side of that patient's midpoint, so that the targets themselves are eight inches apart.

I then tell the patient that when I say "black" he is to look at the black target and when I say "white" he is to look at the white target. I tell him not to look at either target until told to do so.

I then have him practice spotting the two targets repeatedly for about a minute. Then I move the two targets to a vertical position and repeat. Finally, I move them to a diagonal position and repeat.

I test the patient with a total of ten targets in each direction, five with each eye, and after testing both eyes together I test the eyes separately.

To test pursuit skills, I have the patient sit or stand in front of me. I then hold a small black target about sixteen inches in front of his eyes. I notice if the patient has to strain to see the target or if he can see it easily. After the patient has locked on to the target, I tell him to watch it carefully and then begin to move it in different directions. I tell him not to take his eyes off the target as it continues to move up and down, left and right, diagonally. I continue the motion for about fifteen seconds and then test each eye individually.

While the patient is targeting, I notice how easily his eye follows the target and how accurate he is in his eye movements. I also notice if the patient stops breathing while performing the test and whether the patient is targeting with his eyes or having to move his whole head to see the target.

This test reveals how well the patient is able to direct his eyes with his mind and how well his mind responds to being externally directed by me. An inability to target can reveal a mismatch between the patient's eyes and mind.

The Preferred Eye Test

This is a test to focus awareness on one's dominant eye. I place a tube—such as an empty paper towel roll—on a table in front of the patient. I then ask her to pick the tube up, hold it with both hands, and look at an object on the other side of the room. She should repeat the instructions while looking at a near object. I do this test with and without the patient's glasses on.

While the patient is performing this test, I am actually testing her habits. I notice what hand she uses to pick up the tube, and I note whether or not it is the same hand that she uses for writing.

Then I notice which eye she uses to look through the tube, whether it is the same hand and eye, and whether the selected hand or eye changes when the patient puts on her glasses.

This test reveals eye preference and tells me which is the patient's more comfortable eye. It gives me an important piece of information for her eye therapy and shows me how to slow her down. (If the patient is racing ahead in vision therapy, a patch over the preferred eye will usually make things more difficult, thus slowing her down. That usually helps the patient to experience things as if for the first time and enjoy life more.)

Prescription Status

In a patient's first visit to my office, I evaluate how well he is being served by his present prescription lenses and how well he is presently seeing both near and at a distance.

This test is performed in two different ways. First, I use a retinoscope, which is an instrument that measures the bending of light into the eyes in order to determine the needed prescription. I may also use a computerized autorefractor to give an objective measure of the required prescription.

However, I find the subjective examination of the prescription to be much more valuable.

Everyone has had this test at one time or other. The patient is seated behind a futuristic headset. I ask the patient to read the eye chart as I change the lenses in front of his eyes. I then ask how clearly he can see and how the lenses make him feel emotionally. It is also important to know how the lenses make him feel physically—nauseous, disoriented, and so on.

It is my personal belief that lenses selected by this process are better able to meet the complete needs of patients than those selected by mechanized tools. I also share a belief with other behavioral optometrists that it is usually best to prescribe the lowest possible prescription for my patients to allow their eyes to work to see clearly. It also helps patients to avoid the eyestrain created from too-strong lenses.

While testing the patient, I notice how difficult it is for him to determine which lens is clearer and how sensitive he is in general to the use of lenses. Some patients will not be able to determine the difference among a range of lenses, while others will be disoriented by the slightest change.

I also notice the patient's response to the "correct" prescription. Does that prescription hurt his eyes, or does he feel comfortable with them? Is the same prescription helpful for both eyes, or does each require a separate prescription? Some patients will literally sigh when I put the right prescription in front of their eyes, as they no longer have to strain to see.

The Mirror Test

For the mirror test, I ask my patient to stand in front of a full-length mirror with her feet about a shoulder's width apart. I ask her to take a deep breath and look into the mirror with both eyes open. Then I ask her, "Does it feel like the image in the mirror is looking at you, or like you are looking at the image in the mirror?"

I repeat the exercise with and without corrective lenses.

I then ask my patient if she feels as if the space behind her changes—grows larger or smaller or changes in any other way—while she looks in the mirror with each eye separately and then with both eyes together.

Finally, I ask the patient to look closely into the mirror, deep into the reflection of each eye separately, and tell me of any emotions that come to the surface as she looks into that eye and how old each eye looks as she gazes into it.

While my patient performs the tests, I notice if she can maintain eye contact with her own image in the mirror. I also watch for any change in expression as she looks at herself, and I notice how all of this changes from one eye to the other and with both eyes. Does my patient's demeanor stay the same or change with each configuration?

This test gives me some idea as to how much a person is in her body. While the eye and brain are universally connected, the degree of the connection between the eye and brain, indeed, the mind and the body, varies from individual to individual. I can become aware of the degree of the connection by the patient's reaction to this test.

It also indicates whether this patient is the type of person who needs verification from outside herself in order to feel good. Patients who feel the image is looking at them often tend to feel that the world is looking at them as well. This is the typical pattern for nearsighted patients who developed their myopia before age thirteen. Farsighted patients almost universally feel that they are looking at the image in the mirror.

A difference in the perception of the image usually indicates an unconscious internal conflict. If there is a difference in perception when the patient wears her corrective lenses, then I reconsider her prescription, because it may be causing her to block emotions when she wears her glasses.

If there is a difference in how old each eye feels, then I test further for disorders involving eye teaming or binocularity. A difference in the perceived age of each eye also suggests emotional disharmony and a lack of inner peace.

You may have noticed that when conducting this test and others, I give a great deal of import to the perceptual differences between the right and left eye. This is based in my training in traditional Chinese medicine.

In Chinese medicine, everything is related or yin or yang, the passive and the active, the feminine and the masculine. This includes the eyes. In traditional Chinese medicine, the left eye represents the yin energy and is therefore both passive and feminine; the right eye is the yang, masculine eye. The right eye relates to the father and to issues with the father; those patients who have strong father issues will often physicalize them with right-sided vision disorders. The right eye is also the more assertive, focused, and action-oriented eye.

The left eye is the mother eye and relates to the relationship between patients and their mothers. This eye is also the more artistic and emotional and relates to the right side of the brain and its activities. It is, therefore, the more intuitive and receptive eye.

This insight into the different energies contained in each eye is a critical component in creating a vision therapy program for an individual patient. Work that stresses one eye over the other will also bring to the surface emotions relating to both gender issues and parent-child issues connected with that particular eye. Further, a balancing of the two eyes involves a balancing of the yin and yang of the individual.

For example, I had a patient who loved to play the guitar, so we included it in her vision therapy program. Because of the results of her various eye-teaming tests, I suggested that she try to play the guitar while patching first one eye and then the other. My patient was amazed to find that she was quite capable of playing the guitar using only her left eye but was incapable of playing with just her right. We included patched guitar playing as a part of her therapy, and as she became more capable of playing with her right eye, the two sides of her brain became more and more balanced and integrated.

In my years of practice, I have found that my patients have profound differences in how they speak, taste, hear, feel, and think with one eye over the other. As the weaker eye develops its skill level, reintegration of the being results.

Assessment of Eye Health

While the patient is in my chair, I also perform a series of tests to check the eyes for any indication of pathology in either the internal or external structures. Using special instruments, I test for glaucoma, cataracts, macular degeneration, and dry eyes, among other disorders. If I find any pathology, I refer the patient to a good ophthalmologist for further diagnosis and treatment.

Along with all this testing, I also take a full history of my patient's case. The questions presented, first in a written form, and later verbally, are designed so that in the process of answering the questions, the patient is already beginning the therapeutic process toward a healing shift in his vision.

All of this information, as well as the complaints that brought the patient into my office in the first place, are then combined so I can see the totality of the patient's vision and his being. The relationship between these things gives me a picture of my patient's patterns of disharmony.

These patterns, along with the patient's personality type, offer me insight into how to help guide him toward greater clarity, comprehension, and harmony—toward greater vision.

I then set to work in fitting the patient with corrective lenses if they are needed and in putting together either an office-based or home-based program of vision therapy created especially for that patient.

And we get to work.

_____ **A Case for Love** _____

David and Judy were engaged to be married in six months' time when they attended a workshop I was giving. During the workshop, I spoke on the theme of relationships and vision and said that all people see the world differently. If both members of a couple can work to understand the other's personal vision they can have greater harmony, both as individuals and as a couple.

Although David and Judy were deeply in love and committed to the idea of marriage, they both knew that there were issues in the relationship that could weaken their marriage commitment.

The primary issue had to do with the fact that Judy's father had left home when she was just twelve years old. Since that time, she had carried a fear of abandonment, especially related to the men in her life. She tended to project this fear onto David whenever he was away from her. She was filled with anxiety until he returned home.

David, on the other hand, had grown up with a domineering mother. This forceful woman constantly questioned her son, breaking into his personal space with her loud and commanding voice. Because of this, David tended to avoid any woman who sought to be close to him. Anytime he felt his personal space invaded in any way, David would either try to back away or just close down emotionally.

David and Judy had already tried premarital counseling and were aware of these underlying issues. Although therapy had provided some tools that they could use in dealing with their issues, they still were unable to transcend their negative emotions.

I gave the two a special exercise. I had David stand in a spot and told him that he was not to move. Judy was to move slowly toward him while using just her eyes to send the message, "Don't leave me."

David was given permission to verbally announce at what distance he began to feel overwhelmed by Judy. Judy started to walk toward David, and he told her to stop when she was about three feet away.

I then asked Judy to stand still and David to breathe deeply and look at Judy. I told him to raise one arm, hold the palm of his hand open to her, and to raise his other hand and put it on his heart. Then I asked David to look at Judy, make eye contact with her and to pull her in with his eyes while working to not want to run away emotionally. And then I asked Judy to convey the thought, "I am loved."

By doing this exercise, we were able to change how each member of the couple perceived the situation on an emotional and a sensory level. This, in turn, gave them the ability to believe that they could change and that they didn't have to carry their past experiences with them into their marriage.

David and Judy continued to work with partnered exercises and they both underwent their own course of vision therapy during the months leading up to their wedding. As the day approached, each felt excited by their newfound ability to live life in the present, unfettered by past issues.

Finding Your Own Sense of Greater Vision

By now, you may be interested in exploring vision therapy for yourself. In the section of the book that follows, you will be presented with a system of fifty exercises (five warm-ups and forty-five exercises that explore all aspects of vision and comprehension) to assist you on your way.

However, if you seek to become unstuck from your own patterns and adaptations and free yourself from a negative sense of being, you must first create a proper environment in which to change.

The first aspect of such an environment is safety. You must feel as at peace in this space as is possible. While in this space, you should feel safe and unobserved. If at all possible, this space must be your private space—at least when you are working with your personal sense of vision.

The space should also be familiar. Vision therapy exercise instructions often direct you to move freely within the space, sometimes while blindfolded. It is therefore important that you are familiar enough with the space to move fluidly and safely through it. If the space is not in your own house, make sure to spend time becoming familiar with it before you begin your exercises; just sit in the space and move through it. Be sure to touch things—furniture, carpets, and artwork—in order to make your understanding of the space concrete.

Finally, your environment needs to be quiet. While working on your exercises in greater vision, make sure you turn on the answering machine and turn down the volume on the phone. In some exercises you will be instructed to work to either the rhythm of music or a metronome, and you should have these things on hand as you begin.

Remember, you cannot create a sense of greater vision; you can only allow it to naturally occur. You can, of course, increase your sense of clarity of sight. Through a system of exercises, you may also increase your sense of comprehension by improving the connection between your eyes and your brain.

Adjunct therapies like those outlined in Chapter 6 may also be required, as might the attention of a professional vision therapist or behavioral optometrist.

You must also make certain investments in order to allow greater vision: awareness, nonjudgment, time, and selection.

Awareness

As you work, it is important that you are aware of how you process information. See if you can locate ways in which you distort information and if you can come to understand how these distortions affect your sense of survival in the world. Also try to understand how your personal defenses have developed out of your distorted sense of reality.

It is important that while doing the exercises you work to stay conscious of your experience and the process. Don't become so worried about the outcome or your skill level, but do notice how you feel while doing each exercise. Are you anxious, nervous, frustrated? Is there any part of your body in which you feel tension? Are you breathing freely?

If any emotions surface for you during a specific exercise, try to be aware of how old you feel when they do. Try to picture yourself at the age and see if there is a time in your life during which you felt the same way that you do during that exercise. Keep asking yourself, "What do I see?" and "What do I feel?"

On a purely physical level, before you begin your exercises, try to become aware of all that is around you, all that is in your environment. Place a chair in the center of the space and seat yourself in it. Allow all that is in the room to become part of your personal environment.

Become as aware as possible of the environment around you in your work space. Don't limit yourself to just using vision; use all your senses in increasing awareness.

Nonjudgment

Try not to judge anything; accept it all with an open heart.

Work to release your judgment of self and to release the many judgments that you have held against yourself in the past.

Can you accept yourself as a part of that nonjudged environment and allow yourself just to be a part of the world?

Work to release any feeling of shame or blame that you are holding inside of you.

Time

As you begin to work, it is important that you decide what pace is natural for you, as well as the number of days, weeks, or months you intend to dedicate to vision therapy. Whatever the pace, try to go slowly.

I have seen again and again that the patients who go into vision therapy thinking they can make huge changes very quickly are the ones most likely to feel as if they have failed.

If you work too quickly, you can only react to the exercises on a muscular level. Even then, it is not an effective use of the muscles for the purpose of exercises. For instance, if you lift a barbell too quickly, the exercise is of little use in building muscle. In the same way, you must work slowly and steadily in strengthening your eye muscles.

More important, remember that there is more to vision therapy than exercising the eye muscles. When you work, it is important that you have reactions and responses. When you work slowly you are better able to observe yourself and how you use your vision as you work. Remember: as Moshe Feldenkrais said, "When you know what you are doing, you can do what you want."

As you begin, it is also important that you have a sense of consistency. Try to work at the same time of day on the same days of the week. Thus, if you begin working Tuesdays and Thursdays at 2:00 P.M., it is best to continue working at those times. While your schedule may sometimes demand that you change your time, try to make it as consistent as possible. Make an appointment with yourself as you would with a vision therapist and then set to work.

You may get the best result by working every day and by doing less exercise at a time than you would if working only once or twice a week. If you work every day, you need dedicate only fifteen or twenty minutes a day in order to see results from vision exercises. (Certainly, no matter how you plan your personal program, you should do the warm-up exercises every day, several times a day. Those brief, easy exercises should become part of your lifestyle.)

Selection

Like the exercises included in the Bates method, my exercises in greater
vision have been created and selected for everyone. Feel free to try each
different exercise. All are safe; all are effective. Also see the Appendix,
"Exercises for Specific Eye Conditions," to help guide you on your way.
But feel free to work with any exercise that sounds interesting or helpful to you.

When you begin trying the exercises, you may choose to do one
exercise for a week or a month before moving on to another. Or you
may need to do three different exercises every day.

In order to learn how you work best, it is a good idea to experiment with different blends of exercises and work them at different
paces. You may find that you will learn more about yourself and your
process when you work with these exercises in a manner different from
the way you usually approach things. Thus, if you are usually quite
organized, approach the exercises with a spirit of fun and experimentation. If you usually approach life without a plan, flying by the seat
of your pants, try working with the exercises in a very organized and
serious manner. Working against your adaptations in life will help open
you up to personal transformation.

As you begin your work with exercises, ask yourself the questions
listed below. You may find that as you begin, you cannot answer some
of them. Return to this list periodically as you work and see what
answers have been unveiled and what answers have changed.

1. How does my vision serve me? How does it hinder me?
2. Am I able to really see myself clearly?
3. What is it that stops me from seeing myself and others clearly?
4. What are the parts of myself that I don't want to look at?
5. What are the parts of myself that I would like the world to see
   more and more clearly?
6. How would I describe my vision?
7. What about myself would I like to learn more about?

8. What about my world would I like to learn more about?
9. How do I observe things in the world?

What You Can Expect from Greater Vision

The exercises in greater vision are not designed to change you. I hope that they give you the opportunity to change the way in which you see the world. In doing so, they give you the opportunity to experience more, feel more, and live more.

The exercises are designed to stimulate your being in three specific arenas related to clarity and comprehension: sight, vision, and greater vision. The exercises in each category begin with the most basic and move onward to the most complex.

As you work your exercise program, the first shift in comprehension will likely have to do with an increase in your level of awareness, both of self and of others. At this stage of work you probably will feel a sensation of expansion.

This part of the process may bring up myriad emotions as well, both positive and negative. Allow yourself to feel these fully and to consciously stay with them for as long as they last. These suppressed emotions should guide you as you work through the exercises. I have found that patients who record these emotions in journals, with drawings, with movement, or with a tape recorder have the most valuable experiences.

Although you will likely not dedicate more than twenty minutes a day to your vision work, be sure to let those twenty brief minutes reverberate throughout your day. If you do this, they can transform your perceptions and the themes of your life's path.

I remember a patient that I once had, a nearsighted thirty-seven-year-old woman. In uncovering her themes, I found that her first theme was based in numbness. She would go numb whenever she had to interact with any member of her family or with those in her social circle. She really was only happy when she was allowed to go off by herself. She was too sensitive, too easily overcome by people and by any other form of stimuli, and she made numbness her defense against this oversensitivity. As we began our work, I gave her the homework of writing down just how many times she went numb each day.

Another theme in her life was feeling unsafe, even when she was in situations in which you or I would feel quite safe. I also gave her the exercise of writing down each day the number of times she did not feel safe.

Her third theme was a feeling of unlovability, so I had her write down the number of times each day she did not feel loved.

All of this writing gave her a concrete awareness of the issues she needed to work with in order to change her life's path.

Trying out another technique, I told her that each time she ate she was to sit for a moment in silence and give herself a new belief system. She was to tell herself that she need not go numb, that she had nothing to fear, that she was perfectly safe, and that she was completely deserving of love. She was to give exclamation points to each: "I am not numb; I can fully feel!" and "I am completely safe!" and "I am loved!"

In working with this technique in addition to her vision therapy, my patient soon found that the numbers she was writing up day after day were getting smaller and smaller until she had concrete evidence that she had shifted her thinking on these issues.

You may need concrete evidence as well to be sure that you are making progress. Certainly, you can mark your trail as this woman did, by simply adding up the number of times during the day that you fall prey to your own patterns. You can also try the following:

Mirroring

Return to the simple mirror test discussed in this chapter, on page 153. Look at yourself in the mirror. Try to notice whether you are looking at the image in the mirror or the image is looking at you. Try this with both eyes and with each eye separately. Check to see if you are consistent in your perceptions and how your perception shifts.

Space

As recorded in "A Case for Love," in this chapter, starting on page 157, experiment with your own personal space by having another person come close to you. Become aware of how this makes you feel when you are perceiving the world with both eyes and with each eye separately. Be aware of any tension in your brow, your jaw area, and around your eyes as you work. Repeat this simple test over time to see how your personal awareness shifts.

In general, we are all working on vision therapy in order to be able to feel better about ourselves in the world and to allow ourselves to move more freely in it. We are also seeking to explore the world and our own lives with increased clarity. Finally, we are seeking to comprehend our world and ourselves simultaneously.

Attaining greater vision will give you a deep feeling of peace and inner awareness. In addition, it will give you a personal sense of freedom. You will move through your life aware of the subtle rhythms of the earth and yourself on the earth. With the two tools of clarity and comprehension—a full understanding of yourself and your world—you will be given wings with which to soar.

Exercises for Greater Vision

CHAPTER 9

Preparation and Warming Up

In the pages and chapters that follow are some exercises to use in your own program of natural vision improvement. These are grouped into four categories:

- **Warm-ups,** which are simple, basic exercises that will prepare you for your vision therapy sessions, no matter which of the other exercises you choose to do. These warm-ups will also be very helpful for combating everyday stress.
- **Exercises in sight** are those that work the physical mechanism of the eye and are used in combating both pathological and structural vision changes. They are especially helpful for those seeking clarity in their lives. Do these exercises on a regular basis, preferably every day.
- **Exercises in vision** are those that relate to comprehension. These exercises are especially helpful if you want or need to enhance your learning skills, especially reading and mathematics, as well as those tasks related to eye-hand coordination. I recommend that you perform these exercises every other day (three to four times a week).

- **Exercises in greater vision** relate to the techniques by which
  the sense of vision, used in combination with other senses, may
  enhance your understanding of your own self—your strengths and
  weaknesses, wants and needs, relationships and career path—and
  assist you in creating a healing path in your life. Because of the
  complex nature of these exercises, I suggest you do them only
  once or twice a week.

In all categories, exercises are grouped from the most basic to the
most complex. As you look over these exercises to set up your own
program, be sure to work from the simplest exercise to the most challenging. To establish your own program for vision improvement, give
yourself time to experiment before narrowing them down in a specific
category or blend of categories. No matter what other exercises you
incorporate into your program, you should always include all three
warm-ups in each exercise session. While you may add or subtract exercises as you feel necessary, it is very helpful, especially as you begin
your program, to have things as structured as possible, performing the
same exercises at the same place and time of day. In the beginning,
you should be sure that you do not work to exhaustion or aim for any
sort of sight or vision goal. Instead, explore the aspects of sight, vision,
and greater vision through your own unique experience of these exercises. Let your goal reveal itself to you as you become ever more skill-
ful in your performance of these exercises.

If you want a full range of vision therapy, you would do well to
start out with the warm-up exercises and very quickly include exercises from the sight category in your daily work. As you master these
exercises, add vision and finally greater vision exercises into the mix.
In this way, you will experience the full range of vision improvement.

Note that, if you wear any sort of corrective lens in order to see
well, you should start your exercise program wearing your lenses. This
is especially true if you wear contact lenses, as glasses will often prove
to be a physical obstacle to performing an exercise. As soon as possible, remove all lenses for warm-up exercises. Attempt all other exer-

cises with lenses on. Then remove lenses as you become more skilled at the given exercise.

Preparing Your Space

As discussed in Chapter 8, in order to achieve the best results with these exercises, it is important that you have a quiet and private space in which to work. On a practical level, it needs to have good lighting, and it should be a large enough space that you can move about it freely without being blocked by furniture or endangered by hazards underfoot. You will also need a table of some sort at which you can do diverse types of exercises. That table needs to have adequate lighting.

As you read through these exercises, you will notice that some require common household objects, especially mirrors. You will also need such other small items as apples and playing cards. Be sure to read what materials you need and gather them before beginning your exercise program.

A few exercises require equipment that can best be purchased from your eye care professional. You will need an eye patch for many exercises, and you will need an eye chart, much like the one used by optometrists, to check the clarity of your vision. Have your doctor order a chart for you, or make one yourself with paper and a felt tip pen.

Preparing Yourself Physically for Exercise

Following is a four-step process to prepare you physically for your vision therapy in order to get the most out of your efforts:

1. **Breathe.** Many people tend to hold their breath when they concentrate on an important task. In order to get the greatest benefit out of these exercises, it is important that you keep breathing. Often you will find that you will perform a given exercise to the rhythm of your breath, making it all the more important that you breathe deeply and regularly. Breathing will also help you to relax, which will help ensure your ability to work to your fullest, instead of becoming exhausted prematurely.

2. **Blink.** This sounds so simple, but many people forget to blink while they work. Avoid staring or fixing your eyes as you work with these exercises. Remember that blinking is a necessary process for your eye health. It soothes, moisturizes, and relaxes the eyes.

3. **Relax.** Try to enjoy yourself as you work. Not only will you feel better about the exercises, but you will feel better physically if you remember to stay relaxed. From time to time, make yourself aware of your neck, shoulder, chin, and jaw, and if you find increased tension in those or any other areas, take a break from your exercise and relax your eyes, your body, and your mind. Note: While I do want you to relax, it is also very important that you maintain good posture. Do not thrust your head forward as you work, and do not curve your spine either. Make sure to stand and sit up tall when you work. Imagine that your head is attached to a string at the very top of your head. The string is pulled taut, so that your head just floats on your neck. Try to keep this image as you work.

4. **Smile.** You will be amazed at how important this is. Make sure that you smile with your eyes as well as with your mouth. Smile fully; show some teeth. Smiling reduces tension in your eyes and in your whole body. Even if you don't feel like smiling, at least try to get a little upward turn in the corners of your mouth. It will really help you to get the most out of these exercises.

Try to keep all four of these physical aspects in mind as you work. They will really make a difference in your level of improvement.

Preparing Yourself Emotionally for Exercise

To emotionally prepare yourself to get the most out of your exercise program, consider the following before you begin.

1. **Commit.** There is just no way around it. If you are going to make a difference in your life using these exercises as a tool to personal development, then you are going to have to commit to working on some aspect of vision improvement every day. Just as you have to do sit-ups in order to get your abdominal muscles tight and strong, you are going to have to dedicate yourself to these exercises if you want to reach your personal goals. Just as it often helps to work with a buddy when trying to lose weight or get in shape, it may be helpful for you to work with a partner in vision improvement.

2. **Control.** Remember that the difficulties you have with your vision may be more a result of bad thinking and of poor adaptations to life's challenges. So it is important that as you work to improve your vision, you remain open to change and are willing to reshape your thinking and your responses to life's challenges. Refuse to be a victim of your vision issues; instead, take control of your vision, your life, and your future.

3. **Reflect.** These exercises are not just physical in nature. They also speak to your mind and heart, even to your soul. Therefore, be sure to take time to reflect, notice, and consider all that each session has revealed to you.

4. **Increase your awareness.** As you work with these exercises, remember that they are not being performed in a vacuum. They are a part of you and of your life. Be as willing to transform your life as you are to change your vision.

Now turn the page and jump into the exercises with a playful attitude. Return to them every day, following the recommendations listed above, and I promise that you will soon see an improvement.

Warm-Up Exercises

While I call these exercises warm-ups, they can be used in many different ways.

First, you should make sure that you do all three of these exercises before starting the ones in the following chapters. You may also intersperse them among the other exercises as you follow your daily regimen. Remember to do these exercises, especially the second exercise, Palming, any time that your eyes feel strained or overworked by the other, more stressful exercises.

These warm-ups are also very helpful in avoiding eyestrain or to offset any damage to your vision caused by poor visual habits. They can be especially helpful to you if you spend your days in front of a computer screen. While doing any sort of long-term detail work, be sure to take a break each hour and perform all three of the exercises listed here.

The warm-ups do not take long to perform. Begin with a minute each, once a day, before starting any other exercise. From there you may want to work up to two minutes or to perform these exercises as needed throughout your day. All three of these exercises are very gentle and relaxing. You will find that once you have made them a part of your ongoing vision therapy, you will likely also want to make them a part of your everyday life.

Warm-Up #1

Deep Breathing

Goal

This is an exercise that will help you to get more centered in your own body. As many forms of meditation are based on the notion of listening to the sound of your own breathing, this exercise, based on the natural flow of breathing out and in, should be considered a quieting of the self and a preparation for work that is to follow. It will also be a great help during times of overwork and stress.

Note that this is not specifically an eye exercise. As you center your being, it will enhance your sense of vision.

Instructions

1. Stand in a good, comfortable posture in which you feel both balanced and relaxed. Make sure that you do not stand with your feet either too close together, which will make you feel as if you are about to tip over, or too far apart, which will quickly become tiring. Bend your knees slightly. Now, inhale through your nose, breathing in completely, and then hold your breath gently for a count of three. Then exhale through your mouth, and again hold your breath gently for a count of three.
2. Now, breathing deeply, enhance the exercise by raising your head and looking outward and away from yourself as you inhale, and lower your head as you exhale. Remember to direct your eyes to look into the distance; try to see an object that is a long way in front of you.

If you experience any form of discomfort, dizziness, or nausea, stop the exercise, sit, and relax. Be sure to record the number of deep breaths you did before the onset of the discomfort. Start by doing as many deep breaths as you can each time you try this exercise. Attempt this exercise no more than once a day. Your ultimate goal is to perform ten deep breaths during each round of this exercise. As you increase your skill level, you may perform it as many times as needed throughout your day—with a minimum of twice a day, in the early morning and before your vision therapy session.

Keep your mind focused on your breaths and your attention centered on your self and the sound and rhythm of your own breathing. However, keep your sense of vision centered upon the distance, upon the big picture.

Modifications

Try doing this exercise in different postures. It is an excellent exercise to perform while sitting or lying down. In the early morning, try performing this exercise while you are still in bed, before rising for the day.

Warm-Up #2

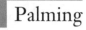 Palming

Goal

The palming exercise will teach you to relax your eyes and to bring them healing energy. It is also an excellent meditative exercise and very helpful in times of stress.

Instructions

1. Start this relaxation exercise with a little friction. Rub your hands together quickly until they feel very warm; about twenty to thirty seconds should do it. Then cup your hands and place them gently over your closed eyes. Be careful not to touch your eyes with the palms of your hands or to press against them with your fingers. The fingers of each hand should overlap and rest gently on the center of your forehead. Don't place any unnecessary pressure against your face. If your arms get tired, rest your elbows on a table.
2. Sit quietly for one to two minutes with your hands over your eyes, breathing slowly and deeply. Just imagine blackness. The more relaxed you become, the blacker the darkness you will see with your eyes closed.

Palming should be performed before beginning any other of the exercises in greater vision. You may repeat it between exercises as needed. And you may perform this exercise as needed throughout the day. Students will find it especially helpful during study sessions to take a quick break from time to time to perform this exercise before studying further.

Look into the darkness of your closed eyes as you listen to the sound of your breathing.

Warm-Up #3

Location, Location, Location

Goal
Try to locate specific points that are high, low, and central relative to your own body. Learn to locate specific places in space and to discover how they relate to you.

Instructions
1. Stand in a relaxed, straight posture with your knees slightly bent. Make sure that your neck and shoulders are loose and relaxed. Your arms should be hanging. Consciously relax your arms from the shoulders down to the fingertips. Close your eyes and take a deep breath. Then open your eyes with your head straight up and look at a point straight ahead of you that is at eye level.
2. As you look at that point at eye level, slowly raise your hands with your palms down and parallel with the floor. With your palms still pointed downward, move your hands and touch the tips of your two index fingers at eye level on the vertical midline of the body (that is, directly in front of your nose) approximately twelve inches in front of your body. Remember that your eyes should stay connected to that spot directly in front of you. Don't watch your hands as you raise them and when the fingertips touch.
3. Now, check your handiwork. Look at your fingers. Are they on your vertical midline? If not, shift them so that they are on your midline. Spend a moment and notice the spot that is in front of your nose and a foot out from your body. Notice the difference between that point and the point that seemed to be your midline as you brought your hands together.

4. Repeat this exercise until you are able to bring your fingertips together in the correct location. Be sure to keep breathing while exercising.

Maintain your eye fixation during the exercise. You are going to want to move your eyes and watch what your hands are doing, but don't allow yourself to do this. Keep your eyes fixed and looking out to a point directly in front of your body.

Modifications

As a modification, raise your arms up over your head, still with your palms parallel to the floor. Bring the tips of your index fingers together at a point that is still on the vertical midline of your body (this time the point will be above the center of your skull) and about twelve inches above the top of your head. In order to check your work, look upward or gently lower your hands, still holding fingertips together, to touch the top of your head.

As another modification, bring your fingertips together so that they are at waist level. Look down to check your work and be sure that the fingertips touch in front of your navel, about twelve inches out from your body. If they do not, adjust them as needed and try again.

CHAPTER 10

Exercises in Sight

The following exercises are designed to enhance your sense of sight. Each is meant to increase your conscious control over a specific aspect of sight, such as eye movement, fixations, or peripheral vision. While all of the exercises gathered here will be helpful to you, some will speak to certain eye conditions better than others.

For information on these exercises and how they relate to eye conditions, please see the Appendix, "Exercises for Specific Eye Conditions."

With the exception of Exercise #9, Pointer in the Straw, all of the exercises for sight may be done without a partner. Some require special materials.

Each should be performed continuously for a period of three to five minutes. I recommend that as you begin you perform them only once a day, two or three times a week. As you become more advanced in your therapy, consider performing them daily. When using a metronome in an exercise, start at forty beats per minute (bpm) and increase the speed as your skill level improves.

Exercise #1

The Four Corners

Goal

This exercise will help improve your ability to consciously aim your eyes and to learn to effectively control eye movement.

What You'll Need

No materials are needed for the basic exercise, but add a metronome for a modification.

Instructions

1. Stand about ten feet from a blank wall so that you can see all four corners of the wall just by moving your eyes (without moving your head).
2. Now, stand in a relaxed manner, with your knees slightly bent. Close your eyes and take a slow, deep breath. Open your eyes and look at the upper right corner. Look at the lower left corner. Look at the upper left corner. Look at the lower right corner. Remember to breathe as you do the exercise.
3. This is the flow of the exercise. Continue shifting your eyes from corner to corner for two minutes. Be sure not to move your body or your head during that period of time.

This is a very simple exercise, yet it does present some challenges. For instance, while you were looking from corner to corner and up and down, were you able to maintain a constant pace? Could you perform all the directions of your eye movements in the correct order?

Be sure to have a conscious awareness of how the exercise feels for your eyes. Do you feel the pulling of your eyes as you do the exercise? Do your eyes feel strained or tired from this exercise? If so, make sure to perform Palming (Warm-Up #2, see Chapter 9) before proceeding to any other exercise.

Modifications

To enhance this exercise, make use of a constant sound pattern by adding a metronome beat.

As you become more experienced with the exercise, try changing the pattern by starting with the upper left corner or the lower left or right, keeping the cross pattern the same.

To make the exercise more difficult, try to visualize the next movement before you make it. Make the exercise more difficult still by performing it with your eyes closed.

Exercise #2

Open and Shut

Goal

This exercise will help you learn to control eye movements from object to object, through feeling your eyes move and through the use of visualization techniques.

What You'll Need

No materials are needed for the basic exercise, although you may use a metronome to enhance the exercise. You may also want to have a partner available to check your work and give you guidance.

Instructions

1. Hold your index fingers in front of you approximately sixteen inches apart. Look from one finger to the other finger with your eyes targeting hard. Move your eyes back and forth between fingers to a slow count from one to thirty. Be sure to match your counting to the motion of your eyes, saying each number as your eye targets the fingertip. Count out loud, clearly saying each number while targeting.

2. Now close your eyes and repeat the exercise. Once you understand the eye movements required, be sure to do this exercise with your eyes closed.

3. Make sure that you are very specific in your eye movements and your targeting. If you are working with a partner, she should be able to see your eyes moving under your lids. Be sure that you know where you're looking and targeting. The muscles of your eyes and your eyelids will tell you where your eyes are pointing. Feel the rhythm in your eyes. Know where you are looking even though your eyes are closed. Know where those fingers are located. Try to be aware of where those fingers are located in relation to the blackness around them. In other words, visualize the rest of the room. Even with your eyes closed, try to know the location of the walls, the ceiling, and the floor. Know where your fingers are in relation to those areas. Keep moving your eyes. Try to see your fingers clearly, even with your eyes closed.

Feel centered in your body as your eyes move and emphasize feeling in control of your eye movements.

Modifications

Do this exercise in different body positions, such as sitting, lying down, or standing on one leg.

Do the exercise to a specific metronome beat. This will help if you are having trouble setting a specific, constant rhythm for the exercise.

Exercise #3

The Invisible Target

Goal

This exercise will help you learn to control your eye movements through physical sensation and visualization.

What You'll Need

No materials are needed unless you choose to add a metronome as a modification of the exercise. You may also want to have a partner available to check your work and give you guidance.

Instructions

1. Close both eyes. Extend your arm straight out in front of you. Now put the tips of your thumbs and index fingers together. Rub them together slightly as if you were holding a very small marble between your fingertips. Close your eyes and point them at your fingertips. Rubbing the fingertips together helps you to locate them. Very slowly, rub your fingertips together and look at that point even with your eyes closed.

2. Now, slowly move your hand around in a circle and follow your fingertips right up the midline of your body and then out to the right or to the left. The direction should be up and out. Move the fingers up the midline of your body and then out either to the right or left, depending on the hand you are using. As you follow the fingers with your eyes, your partner should be able to see your eyes moving under your eyelids.

3. Ask yourself these questions: Do I know where I am looking even with my eyes closed? Do I know where my eyes are pointing? Can my muscles tell me where I am looking? Try to feel where your eyes are pointing even though you cannot see directly. Check your work by opening your eyes from time to time. Do you have to make any kind of adjustment or movement to pick up the fixation of the fingertips, or were you right on target?

4. Now let your hand go around just in a half circle. The direction of the movement is up and out. Move your hand up the midline of your body, then out, then back down again. Then repeat. When one arm gets a little tired, relax and try the exercise with the other arm. Make sure to keep your eyes closed throughout, unless you are checking your work.

5. Now that you know where you are targeting, even with your eyes closed, try to be aware of how far away you're looking. Be aware

that you are not just looking along a line of sight, but also at a spe-cific distance, which should be approximately twenty-five inches from your eyes. Feel this in your muscles. Feel this in your eyes.

6. Now become aware that your target in space also has a relation-ship with the rest of your body. Feel the location of those finger-tips in relation to your back, hips, knees, and feet. Feel how this relationship changes as you continue to follow your fingertips. Keep your arm extended. Keep your elbow straight as you do this.

Try to feel centered in your body as your eyes are moving and to feel in control of your eye movements.

Modifications

Do this exercise in different positions; for example, sitting or stand-ing on one foot.

Do the exercise to the beat of a metronome.

Exercise #4

Head Rotations

Goal

Where the exercises above have you try to fixate on a moving target, this exercise changes the equation by having your target stationary and your head moving. Try to improve your ability to keep both eyes fix-ated on an object while your head is moving.

Instructions

1. Stand in a relaxed posture. Look around the room and locate an object about eye level and at least five feet away. Then stand to fully face that object.

2. Aim both your eyes accurately on that target. Now, begin to slowly

rotate the head from side to side, keeping your eyes targeted hard on the object. If your eyes drift off the target, begin the exercise over again.

3. Once you have mastered the movement side to side, move your head up and down and diagonally as well, all the while targeting the object. Make sure that every time your eyes move even slightly off the target you begin the exercise over again.

Make sure that you keep your eyes tightly targeted throughout the entire exercise and that your target not only stays in sight but is clear and single the whole time. Should the target appear blurry or double at any time, start the exercise over again.

Also be aware of how your neck muscles feel while performing this exercise. Should your muscles feel tight or stressed in any way, stop the exercise, relax, and perform Deep Breathing (Warm-Up #1; see Chapter 9) before continuing.

Modifications

After you have mastered the basic exercise, add additional targets to increase the level of difficulty, such as targets to the right and left of your head and targets above and below eye level.

Exercise #5

Thumb Pursuits

Goal

This exercise will help improve your control of your eye movements.

What You'll Need

You will need an eye patch for the basic exercise, and you may use a metronome as a modification.

Instructions

1. Stand up straight. Cover your left eye with an eye patch. Hold your right hand in front of your face. Clench your fingers into a fist and stick your thumb straight up. Look at your thumb. Begin to slowly move it in a random pattern, up, down, near, and far. Work to keep your thumb in clear focus as you move it. As you do this, observe your thumb and the rest of the room.

2. Notice what happens to your thumb as you perform this exercise. Does it stay in clear focus as it moves about, particularly as it moves in and out, toward and away from you? Does it remain the same size as it moves in and out?

3. Notice what happens to the rest of the room. Is it in clear focus throughout or does it blur at any point in the exercise? What difference does the position of your thumb make to the clarity of your image of the rest of the room? What happens to the clarity of the rest of the room as you try to see your thumb clearly when it moves close to you? See if you can hold your image of the room and your image of your own thumb in focus at the same time. Can you?

4. Now check to see how clearly you can see your thumb. Ask yourself what you mean when you say that you can see your thumb clearly. Can you see the grain in your thumbnail? Can you see any dirt under your thumbnail?

5. Does your thumb change size at all? If so, at what point in the exercise and in what position in relation to your eyes does it change? Does it get bigger or smaller or both? Ask yourself what you can do to keep your thumb the same size.

6. Check to see if changing your posture can change the clarity of your thumb. Does standing in a different posture make your thumb clearer through a wider range of movement? Does standing in a slumped posture make your thumb more blurred? Does posture affect how you perceive the rest of the room?

7. Now switch eyes and repeat the exercise.

Try to feel centered in your body as you exercise as well as in control of your eyes' efforts as they strive for clarity.

Modification
Do the exercise to the beat of a metronome.

Exercise #6

Pretty Bubbles

Goal
This is an excellent whole-body exercise for you if you need to improve your targeting skills and if you seek clarity in everyday life.

What You'll Need
You'll need soap bubbles with a blowing wand, a spoon, and an eye patch.

Instructions
1. Starting with just a few bubbles at a time, blow some soap bubbles and step on them as they touch the floor.
2. After you have mastered mashing the bubbles on the floor, try to catch the bubbles in your hand as they float in the air.
3. Now, try to catch the soap bubbles on a spoon without popping them.
4. Once you have mastered the basics of this exercise, add an eye patch and work with each of your eyes individually.

Try to be aware of the whole room as you do this exercise and notice how your position relates to everything else in the room. If you become physically tired or feel overwhelmed by this exercise, be sure to sit and relax before continuing.

Modification
Increase the level of difficulty by increasing the number of bubbles present at one time.

Exercise #7

Number, Please

Goal

This is an exercise in vision and organization. It will help you to improve your ability to move your eyes accurately and to consciously control what you are seeing and how you are seeing it.

What You'll Need

You will need a pack of index cards and a pencil. You may use a metronome as a modification of the exercise.

Instructions

1. Write the numbers one through ten on ten index cards, one number on each card. Write the numbers as large as possible.
2. Randomly place the cards around the room. Tape them to the wall or to pieces of furniture. Keep the cards at or near eye level.
3. Now look around the room and find the location of each number. Starting with number one, look directly at the number and call its name out loud. At the same time, do the following:

    Look directly at the number, focusing hard and seeing the number as clearly as possible.

    Point with your dominant hand (the hand you write with) directly at the number card.

    Hold the image of the number in clear focus and continue pointing at the number for the count of five.

    Lower hand slowly to your side.

4. Continue through the sequence of numbers in order, following the same list of commands.

Before beginning the exercise, close your eyes and visualize the whole room. As this is an exercise in visual organization, try to clearly remember where each number is before you find it in the room. Be sure to change the placement of the cards every day.

Modifications

Set a metronome beat. Move through the whole exercise to the beat of the metronome. Speak and move only with the beat. If you lose the beat in your mind, start the exercise over from the beginning.

Place the cards at all different heights and distances around the room. Place some numbers on the floor or ceiling.

Begin the exercise with your eyes closed. Visualize the location of the number one card before opening your eyes. Close your eyes before you move on to number two, and so forth. Visualize each number and its location before opening your eyes. Try to see the numbers with your eyes closed.

Exercise #8

Letter Reading

Goal

This is an exercise that will greatly increase your conscious control of your eyes. It will improve your ability to scan objects accurately.

What You'll Need

You will need an eye patch for this exercise. I also recommend that you use a metronome as a modification.

Instructions

1. Below are five groups of letters. In this exercise, you will use these groups in various ways, looking at specific letters from within each group. Use both eyes. Begin with the easiest group of letters (the largest) and perform the following tasks:

   - Read each letter from left to right.
   - Read each letter from right to left.
   - Read every second letter from left to right.
   - Read every third letter from left to right.

T G F I E J K B M W Q O P S K A U W C Z P D J O I S W V M B E K P L K

g j e c o e k q d v p e k a x l z I c t h s w I v m q e y a z m r p e k s x p r y

qwertyuiopasdfghjklzxcvbnmghuytdewskoibvasedrfthukoplmkjnhbgvfcdxszazaewxrvtbunimopve

Plikoujyh gtfr edwsxzcgbumg kepqkudsncxyxwjuyen e nwsis dje eeurndgh wqmvoisnkz ji

Qazswesqaxf trygbvfyhbn njuikmolkmu vyiijekmxmeooplikmnjuhb cfr bhgtyrcxdewsqazpli mk
Plokm njiuhygtvfrdsdx srwfsnue wytshy drtyybciqmsgqxokmryqaikrmpos ncyeghdneis lowjsmepzg

2. Now repeat the exercise with just your right eye by putting a patch over the left.

3. Then repeat the exercise with your left eye by putting a patch over the right.

Make sure that you stay relaxed as you perform this exercise. Hold the book with both arms at an easy reading distance in front of you. Make sure that you continue to breathe deeply while performing the exercise. Keep your body relaxed and motionless as you work, moving only your eyes. Concentrate on the exercise. Be aware of your thinking. If your mind drifts, start the exercise over.

Modification
Having the background rhythm of a metronome is very helpful to this exercise. Keep your eye motions in rhythm with the metronome.

Exercise #9

Pointer in the Straw

Goal
This exercise will help improve your ability to accurately target with each eye and to localize objects at similar points in space.

What You'll Need
You will need a drinking straw, a pointer of some sort (for example, a Pick Up stick), and an eye patch. You will need to work with a partner for this exercise.

Instructions
1. As with the previous exercise, you will use the eye patch on each eye separately as well as using both eyes at the same time. Begin the exercise by covering your left eye with a patch. Stand in a relaxed manner. Pick up and hold the pointer. Be sure to hold it

about two inches from the end you will be using, rather than in the middle or the far end.

2. Your partner stands about two to three feet away from you. Your partner holds the straw still, fifteen to eighteen inches away, with an open end pointing toward you. Now try to insert the pointer into the straw.

3. Make sure you direct the pointer into the straw visually rather than by feeling around the edges of the straw. If you miss the opening, pull your hand back and try again. Remember to move slowly and steadily and to keep breathing while performing the exercise.

4. After every correct insertion, your partner moves the straw to another position. Positions may vary in terms of height and angle toward you. Remember to hold your head still and use your eyes to guide you.

5. Repeat the exercise with the right eye patched. Finally, perform the exercise with both eyes open at the same time. Be sure to feel centered in your body before making the visual judgment and moving your pointer toward the straw.

Modifications

If this exercise is too difficult, use an empty paper towel roll and insert your finger or a pencil instead of a pointer into the open end of the roll. As this task becomes easier, roll up a piece of paper and insert the tip of the pointer into the open end of the tube, gradually reducing the size of the hole until you get to the size of the hole in the straw.

Exercise #10

Explosions

Goal

This exercise will help you learn to relax your seeing.

P L T N D H C O

H V C Z E L S N

T U V P R U Z H

F D N B C T V F

C Y R S P E O C

E O T D L S N B

B R P E Z O D C

A X F S P D O T

What You'll Need
You will need the letter chart above for this exercise.

Instructions

1. Stand in a relaxed posture at least ten feet from the chart. Make sure that you stand far enough away that the letters are slightly blurry.

2. Close your eyes tight. Let your arms fall loosely at your sides, but clench your hands into tight fists. Really squeeze both your eyes and your hands and hold them tight. Now open your eyes and hands

wide and inhale deeply through your nose, avoiding the intense
desire to blink. Hold your eyes, especially your eyelids, and hands
tense and exhale through your mouth.

3. Look *toward* the letters on the chart but not *at* the letters. Make
   yourself aware of the background behind them. Focus on the white
   background, looking as if it were some distance behind the letters.
   Do not look hard at the letters. Look "easy."

4. Now, with this easy look, read the letters out loud in a nice, easy
   manner. Notice how clear or blurry the letters are. Notice the
   whole picture of the chart as you read.

In this exercise, it is important that you do not try to make yourself see clearly. This is not an exercise in clarity or hard focus. This is
an exercise in accepting the periphery, the context of the image.

Modification

To change your experience of this exercise, hold both the tension and
the relaxation phases for longer periods of time.

Exercise #11

Near and Far

Goal

This is an exercise that will help you improve your ability to focus
and to see clearly. It will also help you to improve your speed in
focusing.

What You'll Need

You will need a pencil with letters embossed on its side, a letter chart
(see Exercise #10), and an eye patch. I highly recommend using a
metronome as a modification of this exercise.

Instructions

1. Place the letter chart on the wall at a distance of no more than fifteen feet away from you.

2. Stand or sit in a relaxed posture. Lift your pencil and hold it horizontally with the embossed letters facing you. This pencil will be your near target for the exercise; the letter chart will be your far target.

3. Hold the pencil very close to the eyes, about six inches away. The letters should be clearly readable. If you cannot see and read them, move the pencil away from you until they are clear. But keep the pencil as close to the eyes as possible while still keeping the letters on the pencil clear.

4. Look first at the pencil and read a letter out loud. Now look at the eye chart and read a letter out loud. It does not matter which letter you see and read or in what order you read them.

5. Continue moving backward and forward between the targets as swiftly as possible, being sure that you target and clearly see the letters at both distances. Repeat this twenty times back and forth. Remember to breathe, blink, and relax while exercising.

6. As you build your ability to target, do this exercise with the right eye alone, the left eye alone, and with both eyes together.

This exercise is all about clarity. As you move your eyes, notice which target is blurry and which is clear. Can you make both targets clear? Notice what adjustments your eyes have to make in order to achieve clarity. Notice how long it takes to make both targets clear. Does your vision get clearer with exercise? How do your eyes feel after the exercise? Also notice if one of your eyes seems to have clearer vision than the other.

Modification

Add a metronome beat and slowly increase the speed of the rhythm to increase the speed of your focusing.

Exercise #12

Newspaper Focusing

Goal
This exercise will greatly help you to improve the flexibility of your vision as well as its clarity.

What You'll Need
For this exercise you will need one page of a newspaper. Cut out one headline (larger print size). You'll also need a piece of cardboard (for example, the back of a notepad), which I will call the divider.

Instructions
1. Place the newspaper headline on a wall six feet away to the left of your vertical midline. Place the newspaper page at your normal reading distance to the right of your vertical midline. Now hold the divider between your eyes. Set up correctly, your left eye will see only the headline and the right eye will see only the newspaper.
2. Read the headline with your left eye, and then read a sentence in the newspaper with your right eye. Continue to alternate from the headline to the newspaper for two minutes. See how quickly you can clear the image of the print as you move your eyes from far to near.
3. Now move over so that the headline is seen only by your right eye and the newspaper only by your left. Alternate from the headline to the newspaper for two minutes.

Modification
Increase the distance between the near and far targets, moving the near one closer and the far one farther away.

Exercise #13

Framing

Goal
This is an exercise in eye teaming. Its purpose is to increase awareness of how well your two eyes work together and to help give you control over eye teaming.

What You'll Need
You will need a pencil for this exercise. You may also add a metronome for a modification.

Instructions
1. Stand with good posture and look at any object across the room.
2. Hold a pencil vertically approximately eight inches in front of your nose, so that it is between you and the distant object.
3. Looking at the distant object, notice that your image of the pencil doubles and that this double image now frames the distant object, with one pencil appearing to be on either side of the object.
4. Now look at the pencil and notice that your image of the distant object is now doubled, framing the pencil.
5. Alternate your focus slowly until you are able to frame both objects easily and at will, then begin to alternate your focus more quickly (in about the time it takes you for two breaths) from the pencil to the distant object.

   For this exercise, you should work on two different goals:

   - Your awareness of the doubling of the image of the near or far target when you focus on the other
   - Your ability to maintain clarity of the doubled targets, trying not to let the framing object blur

Modifications

Move the pencil toward and away from you. Notice if this causes any changes in size of either target.

As always, you may use a metronome to set a beat as you alternate your vision. Experiment with the speed of the metronome to make the exercise harder or easier.

Exercise #14

Hot Dog

Goal

This is another exercise in eye teaming. Do it in a relaxed manner and it will improve your ability to use both of your eyes at the same time.

Instructions

1. Hold both your hands about eight inches from your eyes. Now bring your index fingers up in front of your eyes, and with fingertips touching horizontally (tip to tip), move them into your line of sight.
2. Look through the opening between your fingers at an object at least ten feet away. While you are looking at the far target, do you see a floating hot dog in the opening? (Note: Do not look directly at your fingers; make sure to focus on a distant target.) After a few seconds, move your hands apart and return your hands to your sides. Repeat the exercise until you can easily see the hot dog. As the exercise becomes easier, try to maintain the image of the hot dog for as long as possible before returning your hands to your sides.
3. Now, repeat the exercise once more, but slowly move the thumbs further apart and watch what happens to the hot dog. Does it get larger or smaller? How long can you maintain the image of the hot dog?

While this is an exercise in eye teaming, clarity is also important. Notice how clear the hot dog is once you are able to see it. Try to keep it as clear as possible.

The size of the hot dog is also important. Notice the size of your fingers as you move your thumbs farther apart or closer together.

Modifications

To make the exercise more challenging, change the distance between your hands and eyes. Move your hands farther and then closer to your eyes.

Also, while still holding your fingers in the position in which the hot dog was visible, close and then open your eyes. Does the hot dog come right back, or is it gone? If it's gone, notice what your eyes have to do in order to bring it back.

Exercise #15

Pencil Push-Ups

Goal

This eye-teaming exercise will improve your ability to see clearly with both eyes together.

What You'll Need

You will need a pencil that has letters embossed on the sides.

Instructions

1. Hold the pencil at eye level horizontally approximately twelve inches in front of your nose. Look at a single letter on the pencil. Keep this letter clear and the image single. To accomplish this, you will have to focus your eyes and use them together.
2. Now, move the pencil very slowly toward your nose while keeping both of your eyes on the targeted letter. If the target becomes double, both eyes are no longer accurately on target and one eye has slipped slightly. Move the target back out until it again becomes single—meaning both eyes are again accurately on target—and then try once more to bring it toward the nose while holding a clear and single image.

3. Repeat the exercise until you can follow the pencil to your nose keeping it single. Also, keep the image clear for as far as you can on its journey to your nose. Note that keeping the image single is easier than keeping it clear. Most people can usually keep the image single for a greater distance than they can keep it in clear, sharp focus.

This exercise asks you to do two things at once. In doing so, you have to emphasize several things:

- Notice whether or not the image doubles at any point in the exercise. If the image doubles, can you bring it back again to single? Notice what efforts your eyes must make to maintain a single image.
- Do your eyes feel any strain in doing this exercise? If you do notice strain, stop and relax. Perform the warm-up exercises and then try this exercise again.
- Attempt to increase your awareness while performing this exercise. While focusing hard on the target in front of you, try to be aware of your periphery, your location in the room, and your relationship in space to furniture and objects in the room.

Modification
Use bigger or smaller targets to either increase or decrease the level of difficulty.

Exercise #16

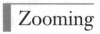
Zooming

Goal
In the course of a day, you take energy in through your eyes and release it to the world. This exercise will allow you to explore the intake and outflow of energy through the use of your eyes and your whole vision

system. You may also use it as a tool to help you get in touch with your personal sense of power in the world.

What You'll Need

No materials are needed, although you may want to use a mirror in this exercise.

While this is structured as an individual exercise, you may work with a partner after you become comfortable with the exercise.

Instructions

This is a two-part exercise. Begin your work with the first part without a partner; do not move on to the second part until you feel confident with the first.

Part One

1. Sit in a comfortable position. Remember to keep your body relaxed during the exercise, and try to remain still.
2. Slowly take a deep breath using your abdomen to support your intake of air. Then bring the air up as if you were going to exhale, but instead stop your breath at your throat level and gag.
3. Stick your tongue out, while still holding your breath back. Try to force the air up into your head instead. Visualize that you are pushing the air upward to your eyes.
4. Now pick an object in the room or use the image of yourself in a mirror and mentally bring that object toward you, as if it were physically moving. Have the object move toward you and then push it past you. Push the object away from you with your mind.

Part Two

1. Look at the same object, your image in a mirror, or a partner, and instead of pushing the object away in your eye-mind, visualize it slowly moving toward you until you imagine it to be approximately sixteen inches away from you.
2. Now let energy come out of your eyes toward the imagined object, really focusing on it as you exhale quickly and fully. Visualize that

you are shooting beams of pure energy out of your eyes toward the object. If you are working with a partner, have your partner share with you his experience as you try to direct energy toward him. (Do not work with a partner until you have become comfortable with the exercise.)

3. On the next breath, relax. Instead of pushing energy forward, allow the image to come to you. Let the object in view be received by your eyes. Relax and absorb the image.

This is an exercise in personal power. It is keyed to the holding and releasing of breath. Therefore, it is vital that you control your breathing as needed for this exercise. You must force oxygen into your head and behind your eyes. It is also important that you keep your body as relaxed and still as possible. Maintain a good posture while sitting.

Modifications

The type of target you select will in part determine the difficulty level of the exercise. It is easiest to work with an object. You will find it a bit more difficult to work with your own mirror image and still maintain concentration. It is more difficult still to work with a partner.

CHAPTER 11

Exercises in Vision

The exercises in this chapter concern perception and understanding. They will improve your ability to understand what you are seeing and make use of images you see. Vision is more than mechanics. We must comprehend what we are seeing and absorb and reshape the image in order to put this comprehension to work in our lives.

For most of us, our formal education ends around the age of twenty, but the process of learning lasts throughout our lives. Therefore, we can and should always be able to improve our tools of comprehension and synthesis, which allow us to take concepts learned and put them to practical use.

Practice all of the exercises in this category for at least ten minutes at a time. You should work the exercise until you feel somewhat exhausted by it, but for no longer than twenty minutes at a time. As you begin, do these exercises at least once a week, working up to two to three times weekly.

You will notice that I have designed more in this category that require you to work with a partner. This is because the struggle for increased comprehension often requires feedback from another person.

Remember to do the Warm-Up exercises (Chapter 9) before beginning any of those in this category. Return to the Warm-Up exercises if you feel exhausted by any of these exercises, and remember to maintain your breathing and posture as you work.

Exercise #17

Child's Play: Jump Rope

Goal
The purpose of this exercise is to use your interpretation of visual information to develop coordination of movement for your entire body. It will allow you to direct your body based on the information taken in by your peripheral vision. (Note: Your peripheral vision tells you about the relationships between objects and space. Your central vision gives you the sense of detailed differences.)

What You'll Need
You will need a jump rope for this exercise. You will need to work outdoors.

Instructions
1. Obviously, you are going to be jumping rope. If you have jumped rope before, skip ahead to step 3. If you have not jumped rope before, start by holding the ends of the rope in your hand. The rope should be long enough to touch the ground when your hands are at your waist. Adjust the rope length by winding the ends of the rope around your hands. The rope will dangle on the ground in front of you. Start by stepping over the rope and back again. Do this a few times to get the idea of how it feels. Use your peripheral vision to notice the change in location of your body as you step backward and forward. Make sure to end by stepping forward again over the rope, so that the rope is at your heels.
2. Next, still holding the rope by the ends, swing it over your head and have it strike the ground in front of you. Step over the rope. Repeat

the swing of the rope over your head again. Try to jump as the rope strikes the ground. Jump to let the rope pass under your feet. Try to keep twirling the rope over your head and under your feet as you jump. See how many jumps you can do without having to stop.

3. Simply jump rope one foot at a time. But to make this physical exercise an exercise in vision therapy, you must not move your head. While you are jumping, you must look straight ahead of you. You must not look directly at the rope, nor should you look directly at your feet. Just keep looking straight ahead of you, directly out from eye level. Use your peripheral vision to see and understand the environment around you.

4. After you master the basic jumping and are comfortable locating yourself peripherally, try to jump over the rope with both feet together. To do this, it is often helpful to jump twice with every pass of the rope. This extra step in between allows you to twirl the rope over your head at a slower speed. Try to spring on your toes and jump twice for each twirl of the rope.

5. Try to jump over the rope with both feet together but this time with a single jump with each pass of the rope. Now the rope will move faster, and your timing will have to be more precise. Make the rope pass under your feet at just the correct moment of your jump.

6. Place the rope at your toes instead of behind your feet. Try to perform the exercise in reverse by swinging the rope backward and jumping over the rope with both feet together in a single jump. This may be somewhat difficult, as it involves your using your sense of the space behind you. Twirl the rope so that it starts at the toes, circles over your head, and passes below your heels.

7. Now, while jumping over the rope, try to swing it from front to back using two jumps for each pass. This requires a change in rhythm, as well as peripheral vision.

8. Finally, try to work this exercise in combination. Try to perform any combination of steps 3 through 8 without stopping. You will, of course, have to stop to change the direction of the twirl of the rope. Remember to keep looking straight ahead. Know where the rope is

at all times by using your peripheral vision. Practicing jump rope will
help you develop total body coordination in relation to your vision.

As this is a very physical exercise, it is important that you pay
attention at all times to where your body is in relation to the space
around it. Be sure that you have enough space to perform the exercise
and that you are able to stay in the center of that space.

It is also important that you stay aware of your body's level of fit-
ness. Do not work your body to a state of exhaustion. Be sure to take
plenty of breaks and keep breathing as you work.

Exercise #18

Child's Play: Ball Toss

Goal
This exercise is helpful in improving your ability to judge the size and
shape of the space around you.

What You'll Need
You will need a table tennis ball and a tennis ball.

Instructions
1. Stand in a room in which a tossed ball can cause no damage. When
   beginning this exercise, make sure to use a table tennis ball, because
   it is easier to deal with than a tennis ball and because it has a low
   potential for causing damage. Your challenge is to toss a ball toward
   the ceiling but not to hit it. The ball should fall just short of hitting the ceiling. This is going to take a bit of skill on your part.
   Perform this exercise for ten minutes. During this period of time,
   keep in mind that the number of successful tosses is far more important than the number of tosses. In other words, if you hit the ceiling with the first toss, you need to take a moment and decide what
   you can do so that you don't hit the ceiling with the second. And

if the second falls two feet short of the ceiling, you need to make a plan for the third toss that will get you closer to the ceiling without hitting it. In vision therapy terms, the degree of skill you develop is directly related to the effective utilization of visual information in directing and guiding behavior.

2. When you have developed skill and consistency in the use of the table tennis ball, shift to a tennis ball. When you can toss the tennis ball properly, alternate between the table tennis ball and the tennis ball to develop and utilize your ability to shift gears.

This still has tremendous relationships to all forms of everyday activity, whether it be driving a car or playing baseball. Driving at varying speeds and hitting a fastball or a curveball are examples of the ability to shift gears in everyday living and are dependent upon effectively utilizing information derived visually.

It is important that you are aware of the rest of the room while you do this exercise. Remember to blink and breathe.

Modifications
To change your experience, adjust the level of difficulty by using balls of different sizes and weights. Alternate tosses among these different balls.

Exercise #19

Child's Play: Checkers

Goal
This exercise is helpful in improving your awareness both of direction and movement.

What You'll Need
You will need two checkers, a checkerboard, and an eye patch. You will also need a partner for this exercise.

Instructions

1. Set up a checkerboard on a table. Make sure there is adequate light for the exercise and that you and your partner are seated comfortably with your feet flat on the floor. Begin by placing one checker on the board. Your partner then calls out which direction you are to move the checker. (Your partner is not limited to one simple direction. For example, he may tell you to move left three spaces and then back two.)

2. You will not actually move the checker but will simply visualize where the checker would now be located, following your partner's directions.

3. Your partner places a checker on the board, and you call out the directions. As before, your partner does not actually move the checker but will visualize the checker in its new location.

4. See how many turns each of you can take while both still remaining aware of where the checkers are supposedly located. See if either of you can actually jump the other's checker through visualization.

5. Next, you and your partner call directions as if you are both sitting on a different side of the board. For example, if you were sitting across the board, where would your checker go? You then go to that place to verify if your visualization was correct.

6. After experimenting with the exercise, use the eye patch to let each of your eyes work individually. Notice if one of your eyes has a harder time with the exercise. Your partner need not use a patch when you do.

Concentration is the key here. You must listen closely to be sure that you follow directions correctly and watch carefully to know the location of your checker at all times.

Modifications

To add to the level of difficulty, work with the checker in front of your partner instead of with the one directly in front of you. This will force you to visualize reverse movement across the board as you play.

Exercise #20

Lost in Space

Goal
This exercise will help improve your ability to see and understand space accurately.

What You'll Need
You will need an eye patch and a tape measure.

Instructions
1. Select an object in the room as a target. Look at that object and estimate how many steps, walking heel to toe, it will take you to walk to the target object. After making your estimation of the space, walk to the object and see how accurate you were.
2. Now select a new object in the room and estimate the number of steps needed to travel halfway to the target. Check to see how accurate your estimate is. In the same way, try other objects in the room and other fractions of the space between you and the object. For example, estimate a one-quarter distance between you and an object in the room in heel-to-toe steps.
3. Now, instead of estimating the space between yourself and an object, estimate the space in steps between two objects. Walk heel to toe between the two in order to check your work.
4. Finally, translate the size of your heel-to-toe footstep into standard feet and inches. Estimate the number of feet and inches between yourself and an object and then between two objects, as described above. Then take out your tape measure and compare the real measurement to your estimate.

Try to get in touch with the internal process by which you are able to estimate space. Does it involve inner verbalization? Is it totally a visual process? Or is it a combination of both?

Modifications

Do the exercise with your body in different positions. This will teach you to judge space from different perspectives. For example, try the exercise while sitting, kneeling, or even lying down.

Exercise #21

String

Goal

This is an exercise in volume. It will help with your ability to better judge the size and shape of objects within your personal space.

What You'll Need

You will need a piece of string about the length of your outspread arms from fingertip to fingertip.

Instructions

1. Stand in the center of the room and choose an object to work with. Your only consideration should be that the object measure less than the length of your string. Decide which measurement of the object you wish to use: length, width, height, depth, or diagonal measurement.
2. Now, while still standing across the room from your target object, ask yourself how far apart you would have to hold your hands so that they would exactly embrace the object. Set your hands that distance apart, holding the string taut between them. Walk to the object and check your work.
3. Correct your work by adjusting the size of the string so that it allows you to exactly measure the size of the object. Again, hold the string taut, and begin to back away from the object, simultaneously comparing the size of the string and the object as you move away from it. See if you can make it all the way back to your orig-

inal location still visually matching the size of the string and the size of the object.

4. Try to decide what adjustments you must make in order to better judge size and shape before choosing a new target.

This exercise requires a combination of peripheral and central vision, as you must move through space and judge details directly before you. Make sure that while you are focused hard on the target object, you remain aware of the room around you.

Modifications
Begin the exercise in a series of different postures, from sitting to squatting to lying down.

Exercise #22

Mapmaking

Goal
This exercise will help improve your visualization of various objects as they relate to each other in space.

What You'll Need
You will need paper and pencil for this exercise. This exercise is best performed with a partner.

Instructions
1. Set up your materials in an area that offers both adequate lighting and comfortable seating. Now, visualize a familiar room in your home outside the one you are in, or visualize your backyard or front yard if weather permits your going outside in step 3. Now draw a map of the visualized area. Make the map as detailed as possible.

2. Describe the mapped area to your partner. Be sure to give complete information on details not included on the map, such as what may be housed in a specific chest of drawers, the colors and textures of things, who might use certain things, and how you feel when you are in certain parts of the mapped area.
3. Now you and your partner move into the room or space that has been mapped. Check to see if the map has appropriate distances, sizes, position, shapes, and directions compared to the actual space.

Work hard to create a map that fully describes the reality of the space you are working with.

Modifications

Try mapping larger spaces. Map your neighborhood or a route that you commonly take. Walk the mapped area to check your work.

You may also enhance the exercise by using different sizes of paper, from very small to very large. Experiment with different kinds of writing instruments and various ink colors.

Exercise #23

The Horse in the Barn

Goal

Like Exercise #22, this exercise will help you build your visualization skills as well as your ability to manipulate objects in space.

What You'll Need

You will need chalk and a chalkboard or paper and a pencil. If possible, have both on hand to work with. You may also add a metronome for a modification.

It is very valuable to work with a partner for a modification of this exercise.

Instructions

1. Make a simple drawing that maps a farm area. Be sure to include a barn and a horse in a pasture that is some distance (on paper or blackboard) from that barn. Give the pasture an open gate. Draw some obstacles between the horse and the barn, perhaps a garden, a big rock, or a building.
2. Study your drawing. Then place your pencil or chalk directly on the horse, and with your eyes closed, draw a line from the horse to the barn, avoiding all the obstacles. You will have to be able to clearly visualize your map of the farm space in order to get the horse to the barn.

Be sure to work on your accuracy in visualizing the path to be followed. If possible, perform this exercise first on a large blackboard and then repeat it on a small piece of paper and notice the difference between the two media.

Modifications

Increase the difficulty by increasing the number of obstacles. Have a partner ask you questions while you're doing the task with your eyes closed. You may also do the exercise to the beat of a metronome.

Exercise #24

Ace to King

Goal

This exercise helps improve your visualization skills, visual sequencing, and visual manipulation, as well as to increase your concentration and organization abilities.

What You'll Need

You will need a deck of playing cards.

Instructions

1. Take out all the hearts in the deck and put them in a pile.
2. Shuffle the pile of hearts. Then arrange them on a table in front of you from left to right, facedown.
3. Turn up four cards, one at a time. Visualize each card and memorize its position. Then turn the card facedown again. Complete this step for all four cards. Now, with all four cards facedown, look from card to card, picturing the image of the card that's in your mind.
4. When you have done this for all four cards on the table, turn the cards over and see if you are correct.
5. If you have identified all of the cards correctly, add another card. Keep adding cards one at a time until you can visualize and recall all of the cards from ace to king.

This is an exercise in concentration. Be sure to move slowly from card to card. Be sure to keep your body relaxed as you work. Continue to breathe. Try to work in complete silence. Picture the cards in your mind without saying their names aloud. See; don't say.

Modifications

Instead of using playing cards, write down the letters of the alphabet or numbers one through twenty, each on a separate index card. Follow the same sequence as with the playing cards.

To increase the difficulty, just add more letter or number index cards.

Exercise #25

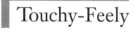

Touchy-Feely

Goal

This exercise uses your sense of touch to help improve your ability to visualize.

What You'll Need

For this eclectic exercise, you will need a bag of some sort; a paper grocery bag will do. You will also need an assortment of different objects like small pieces of wood, coins, fruit, pencils, children's toys, and so forth. You should have about a dozen objects for the exercise.

It may be helpful to have a partner to work with you for a modification of this exercise.

A blindfold may also be useful.

Instructions

1. Place the assortment of objects in the bag. Then, without looking, put your hand in the bag and hold one of the objects. If you have trouble concentrating on the exercise, use a blindfold. Feel the object in your hand. Can you visualize it?

2. Try to visualize the object as solid. Remember, while this exercise resembles a children's game, the goal is not to simply identify the object but to fully and completely visualize it. Can you feel both the left and right side at the same time? Can you feel the top and bottom at the same time?

3. Now, with eyes still closed, take the object out of the bag. Hold the object with both hands. Try to be aware of both your hands touching the object at the same time. Try to be aware of your whole body at the same time you are holding the object and continuing to visualize it. Try to feel the midline of your body as you stand or sit there holding the object. Try to experience the whole object, so that you can feel your relationship to that object.

4. Now, open your eyes and look at the object. Compare how the object felt with the way it now looks. Notice how your relationship with the object changes through the use of your sense of sight.

This is an exercise that will allow you to look at the objects used more completely after the exercise, when your emotions and your sense of touch help to inform you about how the object looks as well as how it is.

Modifications

Use a partner. Have her choose the objects for you and put them in the bag so that you will not see them before you begin. Your partner should be aware that the object of the exercise is not to trick you in any way but to help you develop your sense of touch as it relates to vision. Therefore, the objects she chooses should be identifiable by touch alone. Change the ramifications of the exercise by having your partner use objects that you have never seen before.

Exercise #26

Go Ahead, I'm Listening

Goal

This exercise will help teach you to integrate auditory recall with visual discrimination. In other words, it links hearing and vision, enhancing both.

What You'll Need

You will need an assortment of small plastic toys or objects (such as paper clips, pencils, or erasers) contained in a storage bin.

You will need a partner for this exercise.

Instructions

1. First, you and your partner both decide the types and number of objects you are going to use in this exercise. Once you have decided, you pick up the objects one at a time. After examining the object, place it in the container. Continue until the number of objects agreed upon are in the container.

2. Your partner then holds the container and slowly names the objects out loud to you. Visualize the objects as he names them, linking the objects' names to their image in your mind. Listen to the complete list as your partner calls it out to you.

3. Then remove the objects in the same order they went in. Place the

objects on the table in front of you in that same order, naming them as you put them down.

As you link the image of the objects with their names, you are organizing auditory information. This means you must hold the images and manipulate them while making visual selections.

Modifications

You may alter the exercise by adjusting the number of objects used. If you are having trouble with the exercise, you may also select the order of the objects and call them out yourself before removing them and placing them on the table in the correct order.

Your partner selects up to twelve objects based upon their relationship to each other. For instance, he may use action figures or business tools (for example, a paper clip, a pen, a pencil, and a letter opener). Work the exercise as before, except that when you remove the objects, name them in order and then find their common link. You can start with as few as four objects and add more as you go.

Link the commonality of the objects to sound instead of to use or content. For example, select objects that begin with the same letter or contain the same vowel sounds.

Exercise #27

The Math Exercise

Goal

This exercise will help improve your ability to visualize. Many people find that this exercise is a bit more difficult than most, since it involves solving mathematical problems.

What You'll Need

You will need a pencil and paper. You will also need a partner for this exercise.

Instructions

1. Before beginning this exercise it is important that you have an understanding of you and your partner's level of mathematical understanding. But this is not a math test; it's an exercise in vision. Your partner presents you with a mathematical sequence. She will say, "I am going to say some numbers to you and also a mathematical process, such as addition or subtraction, that I want you to follow with the numbers to give me the solution to the problem."

2. Your partner then begins the exercise with a simple problem, saying, for example, "One, two, four. Add them," or "Seven plus eight plus fifteen plus one equals what?" Gradually your partner will present you with longer series of instructions. It is important that you visualize each number in the sequence and each mathematical function in your mind's eye. By doing so, you will solve each one as presented to you.

Carefully listen and see the numbers in your mind's eye, computing on an internal chalkboard so that you can save the answer for the next step in the computation. At all times, attempt to make this a visual process. Do not say the numbers to yourself.

Modifications

Raise the level of difficulty. Feel free to mix and match mathematical activities by having your partner instruct you to both add and subtract, for instance, in the same sequence of numbers. Be sure that you give positive reinforcement and encouragement to each other.

Exercise #28

3-D Tic-Tac-Toe

Goal

This exercise helps develop your ability to visualize three dimensions.

What You'll Need

You will need some paper and pencils. You may also want to use an eye patch for a modification. You will need a partner for this exercise.

Instructions

1. Draw three tic-tac-toe patterns lined up one in front of the other in perspective on a sheet of paper.

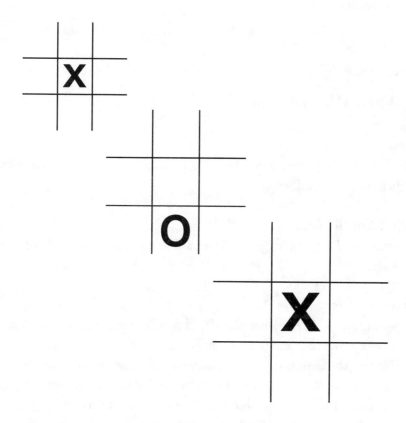

2. Think of the patterns as being lined up like three telephone poles in space, one in front of the other. Visualize your drawing as an actual three-dimensional object.

3. You and your partner play tic-tac-toe in all three at the same time, using all possible levels and alignments.

   Be sure to work to increase your ability to visualize the blocking and winning moves simultaneously in all three dimensions.

Modifications
Using an eye patch, do the exercise with each eye separately and both eyes together.

Exercise #29

Word Wizard Anagrams

Goal
This exercise improves your ability to visualize and to work with both verbal and visual information.

What You'll Need
You will need a set of anagram or Scrabble tiles and a partner for this exercise.

Instructions
1. Spread out all of the letter tiles facedown. You and your partner each choose seven tiles and place them faceup on the table in front of you. Each person then tries to use as many tiles as possible to make a word.
2. Place the completed words in the center of the table. Once there, the letter tiles are available for the other person to move around and use to make new words. As you both work, replenish your tiles so that you both have seven tiles at all times. As you place words on the table, you may add letters to them from your pile in order to make new words. You and your partner should work at visualizing the exercise.

Modifications

Practice your visual manipulation skills by changing the position of the letters only conceptually rather than actually touching and rearranging them. To do so, you both select the first seven tiles and place them faceup in the center of the table. Then you and your partner each select seven tiles and turn them faceup in front of you. Looking at the center tiles, you name a word that you are making from as many of the seven letters as possible. That becomes the focus word for the game. Then your partner looks at his own letters and tries to add one or more letters to that focus word, forming a new word or words. You then work off of your partner's creation. You both continue to add more of your tiles into the mix as needed, without ever physically touching them. See if you can use all twenty-one tiles to create a word tree in your mind's eye.

Increase the difficulty by adding to the number of tiles used.

Exercise #30

The Secret Letter Anagrams

Goal
This is another exercise using visualization as a tool for comprehension.

What You'll Need
You will need a set of anagram or Scrabble tiles.
You will need a partner for this exercise.

Instructions
1. Begin by placing twenty letter tiles faceup in the center of a table between you and your partner.
2. You each now draw a "secret letter." This secret letter can be used at any time and in combination with letters in the center to make a word.

3. Now, you both begin to form words of at least four letters from the pile in the center of the table. Again, this is a conceptual exercise in which you never touch the tiles; you visualize the words as you say them. Once a tile is used, it cannot be used again. As the number of words increases and the remaining tiles dwindle, you may use your secret letters at any time to make a word. As you or your partner use this tile, turn it over to show the other the identity of the secret letter.

4. Play this exercise competitively. Score a point for each word created. You or your partner can use a secret letter to combine with an already existing word in order to steal that word and the point for that word.

Concentration is the key. As more words are added, it is important that both you and your partner work hard to visualize the words and to remember the tiles used.

Modifications

This exercise can be modified by the number of tiles used. Work to see if you can ultimately use the entire set of letters in the center of the table. You may also use up to five secret letters.

Exercise #31

Change of Mind, Change of View

The exercise was adapted from *Seeing with the Mind's Eye* by Dr. Michael Samuels, M.D., and is used with permission.

Goal

In this important exercise you will learn to look at common objects and to shift their emotional and intellectual meaning as you shift your consideration of them. This is an exercise not only of vision but also of viewpoint.

What You'll Need
As written, the exercise calls for an apple, but any common object from around the house will do.

Instructions
1. Look at an apple. Look at it as something to be eaten. You might imagine how the apple tastes, whether it is a variety you especially like, whether it is fresh or not. Now think of yourself as a very hungry person, perhaps so hungry that the apple represents survival.
2. Just as you become a hungry person, ready to bite into the apple, shift your viewpoint to that of an artist painting a picture of the apple. Become aware of the color of the apple, the texture, the light that is striking the apple, and how difficult or easy it will be to paint it.
3. As you become ready to pick up your brush, shift rapidly to the point of view of a worm eating its way through the apple.
4. Shift again to the point of a migrant worker, picking the apple.
5. Now shift to the viewpoint of a small child, bobbing for the apple in a tub of water.

Each time your viewpoints change, you must work to become aware of different aspects of the apple and of different meanings that the object holds. Experiencing this process and coming to understand it will help you to break free of your habitual ways of seeing familiar objects. You will gain greater control over the associations that you unconsciously bring to everyday life.

Work through this exercise slowly, and let your mind float from emotion to emotion. As you become more familiar with the exercise, work hard to visualize the many different hands that may have touched the object on its way to you and the emotions of the persons whose hands have helped bring it to you.

Modifications
To enhance the exercise, work for specific emotional results. Ask yourself under what circumstances you might hate the object or love it. For

example, try being Snow White's poisoned apple. Create the emotions within yourself as a result of visually recognizing the object.

Exercise #32

Vision and Art

Goal

This next exercise will help you notice the details and to simply pay attention to life around you and to the tasks at hand. Further, it will assist you in becoming a part of the creative process.

What You'll Need

First, you will need to find some sort of artwork. You may wish to copy a line drawing or painting from an art book. You may want to use a photograph from a magazine. Even an advertisement will do. You will need paper and a pencil. You may also choose to use an eye patch as a modification of this exercise.

Instructions

1. Place the drawing or photo in front of you so that you can see it easily. Before beginning the exercise, be sure you are seated comfortably in an area with adequate light. You may want to start with a fairly simple picture or line drawing. In time, as you become more familiar with this exercise, you may want to use more complex designs.

2. Start by simply looking at the drawing you have chosen. Study it. Then cover it with a piece of paper so that you can see only the bottom of the picture. (Note: If the paper you are using allows you to still see the original underneath, use several sheets of paper, one on top of the other, until you are completely blocking out the picture below. This is an exercise in memory and visualization, not in tracing.)

3. Drawing only on the piece of paper covering the picture, try to restore the image to its full, original shape by filling in what is blocked by your piece of paper.
4. When you are done, compare your line drawing to the original and see how successfully you have re-created the original.

Be aware of where your mind travels as you do this exercise. Can you concentrate on what is in front of you, or does your mind race ahead to complete the task while your hands work more slowly? Try to coordinate the efforts between eyes and hands.

Modifications

There are many ways to modify this exercise. You may want to work with an eye patch to see how each eye alone completes this task. Or you may want to turn the picture you are copying in different directions before you work. Try working upside down, sideways, or on the diagonal.

Most important, after you have worked a while on this exercise, change the goal of the exercise entirely. Once you have studied the picture and then covered half of it, simply draw whatever lines and shapes occur to you and complete your part of the picture not from your memory or study of it but from your own creative impulse. Then uncover the picture and compare your own creative impulse with that of the original artist.

CHAPTER 12

Exercises in Greater Vision

Y ou will notice that the exercises in this chapter have a more meditative structure than those in the previous sections. The reason for this is that you are now working with the spiritual aspects of vision and with enlarging and enhancing your sense of self.

Exercises #33 through #36 that follow work with awareness and will help you get more in touch with all the aspects of your environment. They will also show you how to properly and appropriately fit into this environment.

Exercises #37 through #43 ask that you use your body as a tool for both comprehension and awareness. You will be instructed to look at your body and image in a mirror and become more in tune with both the reality of your physical nature and the deeper spiritual reality that is held within. In these exercises, we will use the old adage "the eyes are the windows of the soul" to help you explore your own soul by looking deeply into your own eyes as they are reflected back at you by a mirror.

Last, Exercises #44 through #50 are mainly for working with a partner. In these you will be asked to explore your own nature—your thoughts, dreams, hopes, and fears—with a trusted partner. Your sense of your personal space will be tested.

The materials needed to perform these exercises are far different from those in other sections. Be sure to have plenty of paper and pencils available, as well as your mirror.

Do not forget to work through Warm-Ups #1 through #3 before beginning work here.

Since these exercises require more time and effort, expect to work for a good twenty minutes at a time. Also, because of the nature of these exercises, most patients have reported that they experience the best results when they perform them only once or twice a week. Since these exercises are geared to awareness and insight, it may be very helpful for you to keep notes on these exercises and how you experience them.

Exercise #33

Walking Meditation

Goal

This exercise helps to integrate your eyes, brain, and body. It will also help to improve your concentration.

What You'll Need

While you will not need any specific materials for this exercise, it is important you have enough space to work in. You will need a room or hallway that allows you about twenty feet by about six feet of space in which you can move about freely.

You may want to do this exercise to the beat of a metronome. Or work with the sound of soft classical music in the background as a modification. You may also choose to work with an eye patch as a modification.

You can use a partner as a modification to check your work and to change the exercise as you perform it.

Instructions

1. Stand up straight with your feet together and arms down at your sides. Focus your eyes straight ahead to any spot on the wall that is at eye level. You are about to begin making some simple movements to the sound and rhythm of your own voice. For the purposes of this exercise, it is important to create and maintain a slow and steady movement to both speak and move to. In order to keep a steady rhythm, you may wish to use a metronome, set to a calm, slow rhythm.

2. Raise your right arm, saying, "Right arm up." It is very important that you match your words to your movement. Do not move without speaking or speak without moving. As you become better at this exercise, match the pace of your words to the pace of your movement. Practice this simple blending of word and action until you are able to match words to motion, motion to words. Before moving on to the next step, be sure that you have mastered this one, bringing the right arm up to the phrase "Right arm up," and the right arm back down to the phrase "Right arm down." Make sure that you put a rest beat between the raising of your arm and the lowering of it. Make sure to finish with your arm down.

3. Now, take the exercise to the lower part of your body. Again, start by standing straight up and putting your focus on a point facing the wall in front of you. Next, while saying, "Right leg up," slowly bend and lift your right knee as high as you can while still maintaining your balance. Hold your leg up for a moment before lowering it slowly and saying, "Right leg down." Repeat this step until you feel comfortable with it.

4. Next, repeat the step with your left arm and then your left leg, speaking and moving at the same time, until you feel comfortable with those limbs as well.

5. By now you have mastered the warm-up part of this exercise and you are ready to put it all together. First move from your position facing the wall and stand in a hallway or a larger space in which you may walk forward for at least ten feet without any furniture in

your way. Focus your eyes on a spot straight ahead of you, as if you were still looking at the wall. Be sure that you are standing up straight as you begin.

6. Perform the exercise for the right arm, saying, "Right arm up." Pause for a rest before saying and doing "Right leg up." As you take your rest, you should be standing and balancing on your left leg with your right leg lifted in front of you (remember to keep your knee bent) and with your right arm straight up in the air (do not bend your elbow).

7. Bring the limbs down. Say "Right arm down," as you slowly move your arm back down to your side. Again, remember to pause for a rest between each set of movements. As you say the words, "Right leg down," slowly bring your leg down in front of you, moving your foot forward as you do so, so that you take a step forward as you put your foot down. (Don't take too large a step forward, or it will throw off your balance.)

8. Repeat the exercise with the left side of your body. Remember to take a step with your left leg as you lower it. Then follow again with the right side, pausing for a rest between movements. If at any time in the exercise you lose your rhythm or your balance, go back to your starting point and begin the exercise over again. Set a goal of five steps in the beginning. You may want to place an object on the floor to mark your target point. You must especially start over if you forget to speak while moving or if you state any incorrect information, such as saying "Right leg," while moving the left. As you become more skilled with this exercise, set your target point farther and farther away from your starting point.

Be aware of the speed while you work. Be sure that you do not move too quickly, and that your rhythm remains constant. Be aware if you make any error, whether it might be in speaking or moving. Be sure that you keep your eyes focused straight ahead of you at an imaginary point in space while you are doing the exercise. Try not to move your head at all while your body moves.

Modifications

Experiment with different patterns, by alternating sides of the body as you walk, or walking in arm/arm, leg/leg movements. See how many different patterns of arm and leg motions you can discover.

Try working backward as well as forward. The exercise works the same way, but the movements are reversed. Once you have become comfortable with the backward exercise, try starting it by moving five feet forward and then reversing to walk five feet backward.

Work with a partner. Have her call out "Backward" and "Forward," at random times in the exercise, and then follow her instructions and change gears from the point in which you heard the instruction. A partner will be valuable in spotting errors. Tell your partner to be ruthless in finding any error, no matter how small.

If you are using a metronome to create a set rhythm, try adjusting the pace between exercise sessions. If you are working with a partner, have her adjust it for you, so that you will not know how the rhythm will change. When you feel ready, you may want to experiment with having your partner change the exercise while you are performing. Have her adjust it gradually and gently, as an abrupt change will be impossible to follow. You may also choose to work to music instead of a metronome. See how well you can work to various musical rhythms.

As another modification, do this exercise while wearing an eye patch.

Exercise #34

Blind Man's Bluff

Goal

This exercise will improve your ability to "see" better without being able to see at all.

What You'll Need

While there are no materials needed, be wise and careful about the room in which you choose to work. A room containing many hazards, like small, slippery throw rugs or one housing priceless antiques would be a poor choice indeed for this exercise.

Instructions

1. Stand in the middle of the room. Look around to see where you are. Now close your eyes. With your eyes closed, try to feel the space between you and the walls. Feel it in your muscles. Think, "If I were holding a beanbag, could I toss it and just touch the wall in front of me? Could I toss it and just touch the wall behind me?" Try to imagine just how hard you would have to throw in order to reach the wall but not hit it.

2. Check your emotions. Does it bother you to stand with your eyes closed? Do you feel in complete control with your eyes closed? Are you sure of your location in the room? Now open your eyes, and once more check your emotions. Does the space that you see seem like the space that you felt? Notice your emotions concerning the room and the things in it. Look around you. Do things look the way they feel and feel the way they look? Does that room around you look the way it feels and feel the way it looks?

3. Study the room a moment, noticing everything in it. Now close your eyes and point to some object as if you were aiming a gun. Open your eyes. Check your work and see if your finger is pointing to the object. If it is not, adjust your position. Then select another object and try again.

4. Now try to slowly move around the room with your eyes closed. Feel your muscles as you walk through the room. Visualize the room as you have studied it. Try to see the whole room in your mind. Try to walk as normally as possible as you move through the room. Know where you are. Then open your eyes and check to see if you are where you think you are.

5. Look at some object across the room. Close your eyes and walk toward the object and touch it. Try to walk normally as you move toward the object. When you have reached the object, reach out and hold it in your hands as you visualize it. Visualize its shape, its color, and its texture. Open your eyes and compare your visualization with the actual object.

Stay centered as you do the exercise and keep your breathing in a constant rhythm. Visualize the room and all the objects in it. Work to be able to move as freely through space with your eyes closed as you do with them open. Try to use all your other senses to compensate for your vision.

When reaching for objects, be sure to move your arms normally. Do not swing them out in front of you.

Modifications

To test your skill level, close your eyes and walk toward a wall. As you walk, raise your left arm straight out in front of you. Stop walking so that your fingers are just one inch from touching the wall. Open your eyes and see how accurate you are. As you become more skilled at this exercise, try walking to a target object with your left arm in front of you and stop just one inch away from an object. Open your eyes and check your work.

Exercise #35

Shadows and Light

Goal

This exercise will increase your awareness and understanding of your environment.

What You'll Need

For this exercise, you will need to work in a room where you can see outdoors. You will use aspects of the world around you. It will, of course, be most effective on a sunny day.

Instructions

1. Look out the window. Look at a tree and at the shadow that is cast by that tree, a bush, or even a blade of grass. Focus on the shadow. Watch the shadows change as you change your point of view, as the limbs blow in the breeze, or as the sun changes its angle. Begin to experience the world as a blend of light and shadow.
2. Go out into the world. Look at the trees around you and notice how they move in the breeze. Now change your focus and look not at the tree but at the tree's shadow. Notice how the shadow of the tree and its branches move in the field of light around it. Notice the changes in the blend of light and shadow as the sun changes position in the sky, as the wind blows, and so forth.

Try to see the play of light and shadow in the world. Do not focus on the details of objects; instead, focus on light and shadow and how shadows change and move as light plays upon them.

Modifications

Next time you are a passenger in a car, try looking out the window. Again, focus on the shadows that objects cast and not on the objects themselves. Let your eyes play against light and shadow as the world moves away from you. Watch space being drawn away from you. Notice the changes.

Try this exercise at night, working in a room with a light on. See how shadows and light blend and change with artificial lighting. Try the exercise outdoors at night by looking at the environment that surrounds a street lamp.

Exercise #36

Look Again

Goal

This exercise will assist you in developing your inner eye and your sense of greater vision.

What You'll Need

You will need some household objects for this exercise. As an example, I have chosen an apple. You may also use an eye patch for a modification.

Instructions

1. Look around your environment right now and choose an object that is within your line of sight. Now close your eyes, pause, and breathe in deeply. As you exhale, open your eyes and study the object. Notice what you see. Identify the object aloud to yourself. You might say, "A shiny, red apple."
2. Now, close your eyes again. Open them and see if you can be aware of another aspect of the apple. You might, for instance, identify the shape of the apple aloud to yourself.
3. Close your eyes once more. As you open them, see if you can be aware of yet another aspect of the apple. You might, for example, identify some imperfections of the apple.
4. Repeat this exercise as often as you can while still identifying new aspects of the target object each time you look at it anew. Work with different objects to enhance your ability to uncover multilayered information with your sense of vision.

You must identify at least one new aspect of the object each time you look at it. The information revealed needs only to be true of the object in order for you to close your eyes and continue. It is important that you do not overthink during this exercise. Look, then notice, then reveal. Give yourself only a moment or two to uncover new information. Remember to only look at the objects; do not touch them.

Modifications

Although you may not touch the object, you may move in any way you want in order to reveal new information. Change your viewing position when you look at the object. Try sitting, standing, or lying down.

Use an eye patch for this exercise. Try looking at the object with each eye separately and with both together. Notice how you see most effectively, with both eyes, with the left, or with the right.

Exercise #37

See; Don't Speak

Goal

This exercise will increase your appreciation for what you are seeing directly through your eyes without having to *tell* yourself what you are seeing through the use of language.

Instructions

1. This exercise requires that you pay attention to your environment. Look around you. Try to recognize and understand all that you are seeing without verbalizing the experience, either aloud or within your mind. Experience the world visually as small children do, before they learn language in order to identify their experiences. Look around you and see all things as if you were seeing them for the first time.

2. Keep working in this manner and notice how you feel as you clear your mind of any sounds or shapes that you associate with language. If you see printed words on any object, look at the letters as shapes or meaningless things. Look through your eyes and respond with

the visual information alone. Do not say a word either aloud or to yourself. This exercise will help you to see the flow of patterns over a period of time. It will help you to connect what you are seeing with what you saw.

Concentrate on the moment, the experience, and what you are seeing without attaching meaning or context to what is seen. Remember to keep breathing as you work.

Modifications
A simple modification of this exercise is to watch television with the sound turned off. You can watch people pass by. Recognize who they are, what clothes they are wearing, and how they are moving. Don't try to guess what anyone is saying. Work to see the shapes and so forth without a linguistic meaning attached.

Exercise #38

Watch Space Wiggle

Goal
This awareness exercise will help you find your place in your environment.

What You'll Need
You will need to work on this exercise in the world, among people, and outdoors in order to experience many different aspects of the world around you.

Instructions
As you move through the world today, notice that it is never still. Everything is in a constant state of change. The expressions on people's faces are forever changing. People's bodies are constantly chang-

ing and moving. Branches move on trees. Shadows differ in appearance with the changing direction of the light, your point of view, and the angle that you view the shadow. The world that you see changes in appearance every time you move your eyes or your body. Try to let these changes flow. See as many changes as you can. Don't judge them, and let this exercise become a part of your daily life. You only have to open your eyes and look in order to see space wiggle around you.

While you work with this exercise, it is very important that you do not name the images. See them first. Instead of verbalizing by using their names, store them in your mind like the icons on a computer screen.

Modifications
Try to find an object in your environment that exhibits no aspect of change, that light does not move across, and that no breeze touches. By working to find things that do not experience change, learn the constant nature of change in our world.

Exercise #39

Everyday Awareness

Goal
This exercise helps you learn increased awareness through a blending of all your senses.

What You'll Need
You will need to work on this exercise out in the world, during everyday life.

Instructions
1. Select any activity that you do daily, such as washing dishes, gardening, or working at a computer. As you perform that task, become

aware of all the aspects of that task, especially as it relates to your senses: what you see, hear, taste, smell, and feel while working. Just notice this; don't judge it.

2. Now take a deep breath and go deeper. Keep working at your task, but let your senses take in more. Notice the world around you as you work. Are there, for instance, birds singing? What is the light around you like? Notice any smells in the air and the feel of a breeze on your skin. Keep expanding your awareness as you continue to stay focused on your activity. You may perform this exercise at any time and in any environment. You may choose to make it part of your everyday life.

It is important that you stay in the moment with this exercise. Do not let your mind wander; do not let any other thoughts or worries intrude. It is also important that you do not verbalize what you sense. Experience the sensation, but do not translate it into language.

Modification
Interweave your senses to see how they impact each other. Notice how, for instance, when you take a bit of food, the sounds surrounding you modify the taste of the food. Gather as many senses together as you can in any one moment and feel how they work together to help you more profoundly experience life.

Exercise #40

Concentration and Consciousness
The exercise was adapted from *Seeing with the Mind's Eye* by Dr. Michael Samuels, M.D., and is used with permission.

Goal
This exercise will help you increase your consciousness in everyday life.

What You'll Need
Choose a few household objects of various shapes and sizes to work with in this exercise.

Instructions
1. Get very close to an object, so that it fills your entire field of vision. Now, move even closer in order to concentrate on a single detail of the object. Notice what it takes for your eyes to do this, to zoom in on a single detail. Let that detail fill your entire consciousness. See and feel nothing but that detail. Let that detail simultaneously fill your vision and your consciousness.

2. When you have become more experienced with this, try to accomplish the same thing without changing your physical position. Mentally visualize moving in on details, as with a zoom lens on a camera. See the details as clearly and totally as before, but do not move physically toward the object. Let your mind do the work for you.

3. Then, after studying the details through visualization, practice mentally zooming out, so that the object becomes smaller and your field of vision takes in all that had fallen away as you zoomed in. As you work to zoom in and out, notice new details in the object. When you zoom in, become aware of the surface texture and small cracks and specks of dust on the object. As you zoom out, become aware of the room's shape, depth, and perspective and the relationship of size among objects in that room.

You must concentrate in order to do this exercise. Do not let your mind wander. Don't translate what you are seeing into verbal information. Experience the object only as visual information. See; don't speak.

Modifications
Instead of having your vision zoom in to your target, enhance your experience of this exercise by visualizing that the object is growing larger and larger. Let the object fill the entire room and your field of vision as it grows.

Exercise #41

Time Line

Goal
This exercise is designed to see if you are ready to flow amid future time, past time, or present time.

What You'll Need
You will need some sort of line on the floor, which you can most easily create with masking tape.

Instructions
1. Draw or place a line on the floor. Stand on the line and face forward. Think about something that you would like to do in the future—some sort of event or a hoped-for relationship or business advance.
2. Take a step forward off the line. Let this action represent a step into the future. Now, stand in that place, the future. How does it feel? Is it comfortable? Is there a resistance within you making that step difficult? Do you feel fully balanced as you step into the future? Let this simple step be the first step toward your goal.
3. Now go back to the line on the floor. Let it represent the present. Rest in the moment and close your eyes, breathing deeply. Then open your eyes and take a step backward. Move into the past. How does that feel? Sense how you feel about living in the past. Does it feel more comfortable to you than the future did? Than the present? How is your present time influenced by past experience? How does the past influence the future? As you stand in past time, try to remember a past occurrence that relates to your future hopes or goals, either positively or negatively. Be open to any emotions that may arise.
4. Remember that as you move backward and forward each time, you must return to the line, to the present. As you return to the line, ask yourself how you feel in the present. How do the past memories or future hopes and fears affect you in the present moment?

5. Which time period feels most comfortable? Experience standing in the place of past time, which is a step backward; in a place of present time, which is the line on the floor; and in future time, which is in front of you. As you move in the direction of least comfort, be sure to breathe deeply and relax. Surrender yourself to the time period of your greatest discomfort. Allow yourself to be open to any memories or hopes that arise.

This exercise can be especially useful at times in life when you feel you have to make some sort of change or when you feel change is being forced on you. Concentrate and be open to your inner dialogue.

Modifications
Apply this exercise to specific parts of your human experience, such as relationships or career. See how your body changes as you move through time and learn how you feel about these changes.

Exercise #42

The Mirror Exercise

Goal
This exercise will give you insight into how you see yourself in the world. This is a three-part exercise; become confident with each part before you move on to the next one.

What You'll Need
You will need a full-length mirror and an eye patch for this exercise.

Instructions
1. Stand comfortably in front of a full-length mirror. Close your eyes

and take a deep breath. When you feel centered, look at yourself in the mirror. Again, take a deep breath.

2. Look into the mirror. Do you feel as if the image in the mirror is looking at you, or are you are looking at the image? If you wear corrective lenses, test to see if you feel the same with your glasses or contacts as you do without them.

3. Now stand comfortably and take a deep breath. Using an eye patch and working with each eye separately, look in the mirror. Ask yourself how old each eye feels as you look in the mirror. If you wear corrective lenses, try this both with and without your lenses. Take as long as you like to do this exercise. Look deeply into each eye and feel the sense of age it carries within it.

4. Finally, again stand in front of the mirror. Use the eye patch to isolate each eye from the other. Look into the image of your own eye and seek to discover the emotions within the eye. Do not edit or judge what you are seeing and try not to experience it in words. Instead, look into the nonverbal icon of the eye and experience all that it has to tell you.

5. Be sure to end this exercise by closing both eyes. Perform Palming (Warm-Up #2) and thank yourself for your work, for all the insight you have gained. Be ready to lovingly accept all the information your eyes have given you as a part of your self-awareness.

Work to stay in the moment with this exercise and to in no way interpret what you learn. The purpose of this exercise is to allow you to accept all parts of yourself, not to judge them or explain them away.

Modifications
Try an aspect of the exercise that has to do with your own notion of space. With each eye separately, judge how far objects in the mirror look. Look behind you and try to notice how far the wall is in the distance. Then check your work by turning and looking and finally by moving and touching.

Exercise #43

The Inner Smile

Goal

This exercise will help you learn to use the power of your vision to improve energy flow in your body.

What You'll Need

You may use a mirror with this exercise as a modification.

Instructions

1. Really look at your own body and assess it. Scan your body starting with your toes, up your legs to your pelvis, up your chest, and out your arms. Next try scanning one side of your body, from foot, to leg, to hip, to side, to shoulder. Visualize the parts you cannot see. Look from your feet to your forehead in the front and then travel down to your feet again. Experience your whole body through the sense of sight and the process of visualization.

2. As you slowly scan, focus on one specific part of the body at a time. Surround that part with love. Give that part of yourself an inner smile of love and acceptance. Be sure to physically smile as you share that gift with your own physical form.

It is vital that you perform this exercise while in an attitude of self-love. If you feel very negative about your own body, return to some of the other exercises in this category before trying this one again.

Modifications

Try this exercise while looking in a full-length mirror.

Start at different places on your body.

Perform this exercise from different postures and positions. Try sitting, standing, and so forth.

Exercise #44

Buck Naked

Goal
This exercise helps you to really see yourself.

What You'll Need
You will need a mirror for this exercise.

Instructions
1. Begin this exercise alone. Stand in front of the mirror naked, with your clothes in a pile next to you. Close your eyes and take a deep breath. Then open your eyes and look at yourself. Ask yourself the following questions:
    * How do I feel as I stand here? What emotions am I feeling?
    * How old do I feel as I look at myself? How old do I look?
    * How hard is it to truly look at myself?
    * What are the differences between how I look and how I feel?
2. Slowly start to put your clothes back on. Notice how this process changes your emotions. At what point do you start feeling more or less uncomfortable? How do you feel about the clothing as you touch it? As you put it on?

Try to meld what you see with what you feel as you do this exercise. Keep the exercise nonverbal, recording all that you see directly as an image and linking your emotions to those images.

Modifications
As different emotions arise during this exercise, reflect upon how they affect your life in different situations. For example, are you shy when meeting new people? Do you tend to wear clothes that are either very revealing or very unrevealing of your body?

Exercise #45

Eye Contact

Goal

This very simple exercise helps you connect with others in your world. You will need to work on this exercise on the street among people. Choose your partner from whoever happens along. (Of course, be careful.)

Instructions

This is one of the simplest exercises so far, but one of the hardest to achieve. As you walk down the street, try to make eye contact with specific individuals. Send a supportive message with your eyes. At the moment your eyes meet, try to take in the emotional message from the eyes of the other. Don't just make eye contact; make human contact.

Be nonjudgmental of the "partners" you connect with. Do not select only those who are attractive to you. Accept all who come along as gifts from God.

Modifications

To really push the envelope, try this exercise in eye contact with things that do not have eyes (for example, small plants, trees, rocks). If this is a bit much for you, instead begin to make eye contact with your pets, with birds, and so forth. Send the same message of support and seek to take in energy from their eyes.

Exercise #46

Secret Selves

Goal

This exercise is an experiment in seeking the many aspects of self.

What You'll Need
You will need paper and a pencil.

Instructions
1. Find a quiet spot and draw a picture of yourself that includes your whole figure and your eyes. Look at the picture, then at your whole body as you have presented it, and then at your picture of your eyes.
2. Name the picture something other than your given name. Put that name at the top of a list you will begin to make. In that list, express all the aspects of yourself—physical, emotional, or spiritual—as you are aware of them.
3. Now draw other pictures and give names to those different personalities. You may want to draw each of these pictures as you have already drawn yourself. Within you there may be a French painter named Marie, a football player named Joe, a scientist named Albert, a chef named Julia, and a househusband named John. Let your imagination work as you collect and create the aspects of self. Edit nothing.
4. Look at the internal family you have created with an attitude of loving acceptance. Think about the relationships between these people. Who works well together? Who competes for the world's attention? Ask yourself how you can help these family members to better work together and be more accepting of each other.

Try not to just visualize a specific part of your personality; allow yourself to feel how that aspect would be expressed as an actual person. Make this image as specific as possible, with clothing, facial features, and other details all in place.

Modifications
Try to walk, talk, sit, or eat like the personality that you are visualizing. Take on his or her personality and name.

Remember to expand the possibilities by allowing your images to be different ages, sexes, and species of life.

Exercise #47

Sharing Personal Energy

Goal

This exercise in intimacy will allow you to share your personal energy with another person.

What You'll Need

You will need a partner for this exercise, nothing more. Be sure to work with someone you feel you can trust as you explore your personal energy.

Instructions

1. To begin, you and your partner stand or sit at least two feet away from each other, so that you are at eye level. Face your partner. You both take a deep breath.

2. While looking into your partner's eyes, try to send a beam of energy through your own eyes into your partner's. Have your partner become a willing receiver of the eye energy. Attempt the transfer for about thirty seconds. Then rest, close your eyes, and perform Palming (Warm-Up #2) if needed.

3. Let your partner send energy through his eyes into your own, and let yourself become a willing receiver of his eye energy. Again, work for a period of seconds before resting.

4. You and your partner work with sending and receiving energy until you have mastered the exercise. Remember that neither of you should be moving in any way, especially not your head, nor making any sort of facial expression. Simply transfer energy, exchanging roles of sender and receiver. As you work together, eliminate the rest between sending and receiving. See if you and your partner can change roles without any sort of verbal or visual cue. Remember not to compete with each other; work together for a smooth transition of energy.

5. See if you can both send energy out of your eyes simultaneously, so that it meets in the midpoint between you. Remember to breathe as you continue. Rest as needed.

6. Now, try to dance with your eye energies as if there was a tightrope between your two eyes. Let the energy float, first closer to you, and then closer to your partner. In order to do this, you and your partner must actively and consciously work together. Dance along the edge with your partner. Experience whatever emotions come up for either of you. Feel the intimacy, the anxiety, the tension, or the love. Remember to breathe as you work. Work with this phase of the exercise for a period of two minutes.

7. Finally, after you have completed the exercise, spend some time with your partner. Share with each other your experience during the exercise and any insights you may have discovered.

It is important that you keep the connection alive between you and your partner as you work with this exercise and that you concentrate on staying in the moment together. If either of you is having difficulty maintaining eye contact or if a fit of laughter ensues, move on to other exercises before returning to this one.

Modifications
Instead of verbally sharing each other's experience, try drawing what you experienced. Draw the energy you received and sent, including its color, the width of the beam, and so forth. Share these drawings with each other before sharing any experiences verbally.

Exercise #48

Personal Space

Goal
This exercise will give you insight into how you interrelate with the world and the people in it.

What You'll Need
One trusted person to serve as your partner is all you will need. You may choose to do this exercise with an eye patch as a modification.

Instructions

1. Have your partner stand across the room, approximately ten feet away from you. You must stand directly in front of your partner.
2. Your partner should begin to move toward you, closing as much of the gap as you allow her to. Give your partner verbal cues as to when and how far to move. Imagine the space between you as your own personal space, and decide how much of it you are willing to give up to your partner. Say, "Take three steps toward me"; your partner takes only the three steps. You may then say, "Take three very slow steps." You may also suggest size of step ("Take three very small steps"). You are in total control of the space interaction.
3. Since you are in control, you may also tell your partner to stop. Consider your own emotional state and your desires before allowing your partner to approach or touch you. You may end the exercise at any time and with any distance between you.
4. Now move toward your partner, with all the same rules applying.
5. Next try this exercise without the person being approached giving verbal instructions. You both take a turn being approached by the other, noticing how you feel as you are being approached.
6. After you have tried this exercise, consider the following questions. See what insights they yield and share the information with each other:
   - What feelings surface for you as you are being approached by the other person? As you approach the other person?
   - Is there a difference when you are giving the instructions as opposed to following the instructions? Which do you prefer?
   - How close can the other person come toward you in both ways before you feel anxious, nervous, or scared? How do you want to react as she approaches? Do you want to run away, fight her, or go numb?

Try to stay in touch with your own sense of safety and self and how that might be impacted upon by the approach of another.

Modifications

Try this exercise while the person being approached has her eyes closed.

Have the approaching partner come toward the other from the side, from behind, or from an angle.

Try having the person being approached sit or squat down as her partner comes toward her.

Use an eye patch to have the person being approached experience the exercise with one eye at a time. Compare the results each eye gives.

Exercise #49

The Eye of the Beholder

Goal

This exercise will enhance your connection and relationship with your partner. Enhancing your relationship with a loved one will enhance your vision as well.

It's best to use a loved one as your partner for this exercise.

Instructions

1. Both you and your partner take off your shoes and socks. Face your partner, standing about two feet away. If you are different heights, sit in a chair so that you are at eye level.

2. Gaze into each other's eyes. Notice if you can easily look at both of your partner's eyes simultaneously, or if you tend to look at one eye more than the other. Look at your partner's eyes as he looks into yours and breathe. Try to see from your heart and not just your eyes. Put your hand on your heart and gaze into your partner's eyes. Feel any emotions that surface. Do this phase of the exercise for approximately one minute.

3. While still gazing into each other's eyes, hold each other's hands and make a connection. You are now connected with both eyes and

hands, both physically and energistically. Do this for one minute. Keep breathing. Feel whatever emotions surface for you.

4. While still holding hands, put your feet together and touch toes. Continue gazing into each other's eyes. Keep breathing. Do this for one minute. Feel your own emotions as they arise.

5. Sit or stand joined together for as long as is comfortable. Either partner may end the exercise at any time. After you have finished the exercise, share what insights or emotional responses have arisen for either of you.

Center yourself in the relationship you feel with this person. This is not an exercise in visualization, so do not add or subtract any sort of emotion. Simply feel what you feel and stay in the moment with your partner.

Modifications

You may choose to keep your shoes on for this exercise modification. Begin the exercise sitting. Look into each other's eyes. Touch hands. With hands touching and while still making eye contact, begin to move together with slow, gentle, palm-to-palm gestures. As you become more confident of your connection, you may jointly rise and move freely around the room, all the while maintaining eye and hand contact. Notice if one or the other seems to lead in these movements. Work to move completely together, as if of one mind.

Exercise #50

Experiencing the Eye-Soul Dialogue

Goal

This complex exercise will help you to become more aware of the deeper aspects of your vision as you become aware of the deeper aspects of yourself. In exploring this exercise, you experience everyday tasks in new ways.

What You'll Need

You will need a journal for this exercise. Choose any kind you like, from loose typing paper, to a three-ring notebook, to a leather-bound volume, but spend some time selecting the right journal.

You will also need an eye patch, a mirror, a lead pencil, and colored pencils plus any of the other objects you have used in past exercises.

Instructions

1. Eat a meal with one eye patched. Observe yourself while you eat. Notice your thoughts and note any changes from your usual mindset. Notice your feelings, not only as you eat, but how you feel in general as you have one eye covered. Notice how the food tastes. Notice the smell of the food. Notice how you feel physically. Does wearing the eye patch make you feel disoriented? Does it make you feel more or less hungry than usual? Use your journal to record all that you observe. Repeat with the other eye during another meal.

2. After you finish your meal, wash the dishes with one eye patched. Is the task changed in any way? Do you feel different emotions from those that you would usually feel while working at this simple task? Notice any changes or any emotional issues raised. Repeat this task at another meal with the other eye.

3. Take a walk outside with one eye patched. Notice how the world looks. Is the quality of your vision the same as usual? If it has changed, note how. Is your experience of the world different while using just one eye? Note whatever emotions arise as you enter the world using just one eye.

4. Do something creative with each eye separately. Draw, paint, play a musical instrument, or sing. Notice your degree of self-expression with each eye. Notice how each eye approaches creative activities. Notice your degree of comfort or discomfort with each eye.

5. Now go back and explore some of the other exercises in this book, using whatever props or materials they require, and work the exercises with each eye separately. Notice the emotional ramifications of these exercises and consider the information they bring you.

6. Connect with a good friend, companion, or lover as a partner for ten minutes with each eye. Notice how you relate to your partner. Get feedback from your partner about what she experienced during the exercise.

7. Go to a quiet and private place and spend ten minutes looking into a mirror using each eye separately. Observe your own reflection as if seeing it for the first time. Look deeply into each eye and remain open to whatever information it gives you. Ask yourself the following questions about each eye:

   • How does this eye feel? What does it think its job is? How well does it feel it is doing its job? What does it consider to be its strength? Its weakness?

   • How does this eye feel about me as a whole person?

   • How does this eye feel about the other eye?

   • How does this eye feel about my mother? How does it feel about my father?

   • How do I feel about this eye separately from the other? Is there anything I can do to help it to do its job? To change and grow?

   • What do I feel in my body as I have these conversations? As I gather information from within?

8. Think and feel about your eyes, both as individual beings and as a team working together. Do your eyes feel like living things to you? How well do you feel your eyes work together for you, and how does that manifest in your sense of self and your ability to live your life? What can you do to enhance your eyes' teamwork and your feeling of internal unity and wholeness?

9. Keep this information, along with all the rest you have gathered, in your journal. Note that your journal is a book that you are creating for yourself, and you need never show it to anyone else. Begin working with your journal by drawing each eye separately and then drawing them together. Do not worry about whether your sketches are realistic or not; simply draw them the way you feel them to be. If you wish, use colored pencils to enhance the drawings. Draw your eyes as often as you desire.

10. Keep daily records in your journal, both written and drawn. Explore how you can record information nonverbally, how best you can record your experiences with the full range of exercises in this book, and how these experiences can create positive change in your life.

Experience your sense of vision and of self in a nonjudgmental way. Try to stand back from yourself as you work, observe, experience, and feel, but try not to edit.

Modifications

Do aspects of this exercise at different times of the day, different days of the week, and at different locations.

Add other tasks to the mix. Explore the ways you live your life and the ways in which a sense of greater vision can enhance that life.

Exercises for Specific Eye Conditions

All the exercises included in this book are both safe and appropriate for all readers, no matter their age or eye condition. However, some exercises are more suited to some readers than others. Here is a list of the common vision conditions discussed in this book, along with a number of exercises that each suggests. As you work to improve your vision, consider which exercises your vision condition might suggest.

Functional Conditions

Convergence Excess

If you have convergence excess, it is important for you to learn to relax and to not try so very hard, both in the process of seeing and in living your life. As you work, remember to breathe, to smile, and to not be too serious. Have fun. I recommend the following exercises because they require you to focus on a target while not getting too drawn in to the details.

Open and Shut, #2: This exercise will help you learn to control your eye movements through the use of visualization. Remember: if you have convergence excess, you tend to overfocus on a target.

Invisible Target, #3: Try this exercise in order to experiment with your control over your eye movements, both through physical sensation and visualization.

Hot Dog, #14: Use this exercise to learn how to relax your eyes while looking at near targets. It may not be your favorite exercise, but it is a good one for you to work with.

Ball Toss, #18: This exercise will teach you to judge space more accurately.

Horse in the Barn, #23: This exercise will improve your ability to visualize.

Vision and Art, #32: This exercise will help stimulate your right brain and enhance your creative side.

Blind Man's Bluff, #34: This excellent exercise will teach you to rely on your other senses so you can orient yourself in the world while relaxing your whole visual system.

Convergence Insufficiency

If you have convergence insufficiency, it is important for you to learn to stay in the present moment while attempting to perform any task. You must learn to concentrate on what you are doing in order to stay in the present moment. You have the tendency to let your mind (to say nothing of your eyes) wander. Daydreaming is your safe haven, but daydreaming alone accomplishes nothing. So it is time for you to buckle down. I recommend the following exercises just for you. They will require you to concentrate, center yourself, and sustain your mind and your eyes on a visual target.

Pointer in the Straw, #9: This exercise will teach you to localize, to target. Remember that being able to locate objects in space is a by-product of a flexible visual system.

Framing, #13: This exercise will give you direct feedback if you are using both of your eyes together or if you have allowed one eye to become dominant.

Pencil Push-Ups, #15: This exercise will help increase your eye muscles' ability to focus as the target moves closer. Therefore, it is an excellent exercise to use to build convergence skills. Perhaps you should stress this exercise as you begin your work.

Word Wizard Anagrams, #29: This exercise will increase your eyes' and mind's ability to attend to a task.

Walking Meditation, #33: This exercise will help keep your eyes and mind focused. Note that it is a somewhat advanced exercise and may be too difficult for when you are just beginning.

Eye Contact, #45: This exercise will help you improve your visual, mental, and emotional focus in life.

Personal Space, #48: This exercise will help you work through your need to protect yourself from other people.

Strabismus

If you've been diagnosed with strabismus, it is important to learn how each of your eyes perceives the world around it. Once you become aware of this, you will then be able to learn how they can work together as a team. I recommend the following exercises in order to build maximum flexibility in your eye muscles and to give you insight into how your two eyes interact with the world around them. As you work, it is important for you to consider your condition as an opportunity to discover previously shut-down parts of yourself, not as something to be ashamed of.

Esotropia
Four Corners, #1: This is a good exercise for you to use to build maximum flexibility of the extraocular muscles in the eyes. Start your

work slowly, as your eye muscles may tire easily. But work with this exercise often.

Head Rotations, #4: This exercise will help you release the tension in your upper neck and occipital areas.

Jump Rope, #17: This exercise will help you learn to integrate your central vision with your peripheral senses while you are moving about in space. Use this exercise to develop your coordination for your whole body, not just your eyes. Let yourself move in a fluid motion, as directed by your eyes. Note that the exercise is based on the information that is taken in as your peripheral vision tells you about the relationships between objects and the space they are in. Your central vision, on the other hand, tells you about the detailed differences between objects.

String, #21: Use this exercise to learn to localize where objects are in space, first with each eye by itself and then later using both eyes at once. This will help your eyes work better together. It will help you to be better able to judge the sizes and shapes of objects as they enter your personal space.

Look Again, #36: This exercise will develop the connection between your mind and your eyes.

Secret Selves, #46: This exercise will help you get in contact with the different parts of yourself so that you can become more integrated.

Eye-Soul Dialogue, #50: This exercise will help you to uncover the underlying emotional and soul issues that sit at the core of your being. Allow yourself to feel whatever emotions arise. My strabismus patients find this to be one of their most important exercises.

Exotropia
Letter Reading, #8: Work with this exercise to build your ability to focus your eyes and mind together in order to better process your information. This is an exercise that should be done slowly, with full concentration.

Pointer in the Straw, #9: Try this exercise if you want to learn to localize where things are in space. This skill requires that you use your two eyes as an effective team. It will enhance that required team-work by allowing you to accurately target with each eye and to local-ize objects with both eyes together.

Checkers, #19: This exercise will develop your abilities to ori-ent your mind and eyes on a visual task.

Touchy-Feely, #25: This exercise is helpful if you need to learn to focus your mind on the sense of touch. In doing so, you'll increase your ability to visualize and to process information, all without using your eyes.

Everyday Awareness, #39: The goal of this exercise is to increase your level of observation and attention in your life.

Concentration and Consciousness, #40: The goal of this exer-cise is to improve your mind's ability to be present.

Eye-Soul Dialogue, #50: This deep-working exercise will help you to uncover emotional and soul issues based in each eye. Wait until you have tried some of the more basic exercises before moving on to this one, and be willing to completely experience and honor any emo-tions that arise.

Amblyopia

If you have been diagnosed with having a lazy eye, it is very impor-tant that you learn to trust the information that comes in through that eye. To do so, use these exercises to put you into situations in which you will have to relate with the world while using various different senses. Along the way you are going to work to overcome the idea that the amblyopic eye is truly lazy or bad. Instead, think of that eye like you think of Sleeping Beauty, as something beautiful that is beginning to stir. Finally, I recommend the following exercises to stimulate and energize your amblyopic eye.

Pretty Bubbles, #6: Work with this exercise in order to ulti-mately have your weaker eye able to follow a changing target. This is an excellent exercise for improving aiming skills in general, although you may find it difficult at first. Don't give up. Keep working, and remember to keep breathing as you work.

Letter Reading, #8: If you work with this exercise, you will increase your conscious control over your eyes. You will also increase your ability to scan objects and to pay attention to all the details of what you have scanned.

Newspaper Focusing, #12: This exercise will greatly help you improve the flexibility of the amblyopic eye. In general, it will help your ability to focus and to achieve clarity.

3-D Tic-Tac-Toe, #28: This exercise will improve the ability of the mind's eye to see and visualize space.

Shadows and Light, #35: This exercise will increase the ability of the eyes to discriminate changes in their world.

Eye Contact, #45: This is an important exercise, as it will help you to develop your skills for eye contact, something underdeveloped in most amblyopes. Be aware that as you work with the exercise, you will likely experience many emotions that have been deeply buried, so be sure to work with a partner that you trust.

Eye-Soul Dialogue, #50: This is an important exercise because it will help you reprogram the belief systems associated with the amblyopic eye.

Eye Movement Disorders

If you have an eye movement disorder of any sort, your experience of the world will likely seem somewhat split, as if your eyes are traveling at one speed and your mind at another. Therefore, it is important in your vision therapy that you learn to slow down and gain conscious control over all the movements of your eyes. Ultimately, you want your eyes to do what your brain tells them to do. The key to your work is that you immediately slow down and concentrate your attention on the tasks ahead. The listed exercises will help you to develop an integration between your eyes and your mind.

Four Corners, #1: Explore this exercise in order to learn to better control the movements of your eyes. Be careful to work slowly and steadily with this exercise and do not work too long or hard—avoid working your eyes to exhaustion.

Number, Please, #7: This is an organizational exercise and will help you organize visually. It will also help you improve your ability to move your eyes accurately and to consciously control both what you are seeing and how you are seeing it.

Lost in Space, #20: This exercise will help improve your ability to see and understand what you have seen. It is especially helpful in guiding you through your perception of the space around you.

Mapmaking, #22: This exercise will help you develop your visual organization skills so that you can be more organized.

Ace to King, #24: Use this exercise to improve your visualization skills, your visual sense of sequencing, and your visual manipulation. It is also an excellent exercise for building concentration and increasing organization abilities.

Go Ahead, I'm Listening, #26: This exercise will increase your ability to sustain attention for longer periods of time.

Secret Letter Anagrams, #30: This exercise will help you keep your eyes and mind on a task.

Farsightedness (Hyperopia) and/or Presbyopia

If you have been diagnosed with farsightedness, you probably have very good distance-oriented skills for tasks like playing sports and driving a car. But most people who are farsighted have difficulty both paying attention and sustaining clarity with close images and with details. The exercises listed below will help you control your eyes' focusing system. They will also help you to stay in the present moment.

If you have been told that you have the condition known as presbyopia, you may also have been told that after age forty, an inability to read a printed page that is within arm's length is normal and that your eye muscles have aged like the rest of your body. Work with these exercises to restore your flexibility of vision and to avoid needing reading glasses.

Letter Reading, #8: This exercise will help you improve the ability to focus your mind and eye on detail work.

Near/Far, #11: Work with this exercise to develop the specific skill of focusing. It will also help you to more easily and more thoroughly understand the image taken in by your eyes.

Newspaper Focusing, #12: Again, with this exercise you work with the specific skill of focusing and identifying what you are seeing.

Framing, #13: The purpose of the exercise is to increase your awareness of how well your two eyes are working together as you change your attention and focus from near to far.

Pencil Push-Ups, #15: Work hard with this exercise. It's good for you. It will help you to increase your ability to sustain near focus.

Walking Meditation, #33: Use this exercise to better integrate your eyes, your brain, and your body. It will also help you to improve your concentration and to stay in the present moment. Concentrate hard as you work. Don't let your mind drift.

Time Line, #41: This exercise will help you better deal with what's going on in your present life.

Nearsightedness and Astigmatism

If you have a diagnosis of either nearsightedness or astigmatism, you tend to show tension and constriction in your eyes and throughout your body. All of the exercises listed here will help you to relax and open up the areas of your mind and body in which you hold most of your tension. As you work, remember to breathe, blink, smile, and enjoy yourself. Let yourself go.

Head Rotations, #4: You likely hold a good deal of tension in your neck and around the occipital area in the back of the head. Head rotations performed with the proper breath support are therefore very helpful. Do them slowly and gently, with an emphasis on relaxation. They are an excellent way both to begin and end an exercise session.

Explosions, #10: In yoga, there is a theory that in order to know how to relax a part of the body, you first have to be aware of just how tense it is. This exercise will help to both relieve the tension you carry in your eyes and bring oxygen into your eyes as you work.

Near/Far, #11: Use this exercise to build flexibility in the muscles that control focusing. These muscles tend to be very tight and very inflexible in those with nearsightedness and astigmatism, which, in and of itself, cannot cause the conditions at hand but can greatly enhance them. Learning to consciously control your focusing muscles will help you overcome nearsightedness.

Hot Dog, #14: Work with this exercise in order to learn how to better use your two eyes together in a relaxed manner. It will give you feedback on the difference between your two eyes when they are tense and when they are relaxed.

Zooming, #16: Use this exercise to learn to let go of tension in both the muscles inside and outside of the eye.

See; Don't Speak, #37: This exercise will help you decrease the inner chatter in your mind so that you can just let your vision happen.

Buck Naked, #44: This exercise will help get you in touch with your inner vulnerabilities.

Pathological Conditions

Cataracts

If you have a diagnosis of cataracts, then one or both of the lenses of your eyes have begun to harden and to lose circulation. The following exercises are structured to help you to rebuild some elasticity in your lenses and to increase circulation to your eyes. It is important when dealing with cataracts that in addition to any vision therapy you may choose to undertake, you establish and follow a good nutritional program. Many times, surgery is ultimately indicated for those with cataracts. Consult an ophthalmologist if you have received this diagnosis.

Palming, Warm-Up #2: Stop and perform this simple warm-up exercise several times each day. It brings healing energy to the eyes.

Near/Far, #11: This exercise will help you to exercise the lenses of your eyes. Concentrate on letting your vision and your awareness gently flow in and out as you work with this exercise.

Zooming, #16: This exercise brings a good deal of oxygen to your eyes. It will also help you build flexibility to the eye area.

Dry Eyes

As with cataracts, dry eyes usually indicate a deficiency of circulation in the eyes. If this is your diagnosis, the following exercises will help keep your corneas moist by stimulating the mechanism responsible for keeping eyes lubricated. Even with vision exercises, it is important that you establish and keep a solid nutritional program. Eye drops may also be helpful. Consult an eye care professional if you suffer from dry eyes.

Palming, Warm-Up #2: This exercise helps to bring energy to the eyes and also increases circulation. I cannot stress enough that you should perform it each day, as often as you like. You cannot do this exercise too often.

Open and Shut, #2: Use this exercise in order to learn to focus your eyes properly, as well as how to blink regularly. Many people with dry eyes do not blink enough. Blinking is vital to moisturizing the eyes.

Buck Naked, #44: This exercise will help you get in touch with any unexpressed emotions that you might be suppressing. Suppressed emotion, especially grief, often underlies dry eyes. Give yourself permission to feel, permission to cry.

Glaucoma

If you suffer from glaucoma then you have pent-up pressure and tension in your eyes. The following exercises will help you to reduce some of that tension. In addition to eye exercises, it is important that you work to control your condition nutritionally and that you consult an eye care professional. Medication will most likely be required to control this condition.

Palming, Warm-Up #2: Again, I cannot recommend this exercise enough. It brings both healing energy and relaxation to the eyes and will also help to stimulate some very powerful acupressure points located around the eyes that can help reduce tension.

Four Corners, #1: Working slowly and gently with this exercise will help bring flexibility to your eyes. It will also help to relax tension in the area around the eyes.

Inner Smile, #43: This exercise will help you to learn to use the power of vision to improve the energy flow throughout your whole body.

Macular Degeneration

If you have been told that you have macular degeneration, then you have a lack of circulation to the area of the eye called the macula, which is responsible for your central, or detailed, vision. These exercises will help your vision by stimulating the macula. Along with exercises, it is very important that you follow a nutritional program, as research has shown that specific nutrients both prevent and improve the condition. It is important that you are under the treatment of a trained eye doctor if you have macular degeneration.

Palming, Warm-Up #2: Bring healing energy to your eyes several times a day by stopping whatever you are doing and palming. Palming will also stimulate acupressure points around your eyes that are of vital help to your circulation.

Thumb Pursuits, #5: By making you focus your eyes on a target, this exercise will help to stimulate the macula and improve your vision.

Look Again, #36: Use this exercise to help you develop a relationship between your inner and outer vision. See how well you can improve your sight through a process that balances visualization and seeing.

Notes

An enormous amount of research went into this book. Rather than list every source, the following are the references most directly related to the information in each chapter.

Chapter 1

Anshel, J. *Smart Medicine for Your Eyes*. Garden City Park, New York: Avery Publishing, 1999.

Carterette, Edward C., and Friedman, Morton P. *Handbook of Perception*, Vol. 5 of *Seeing*. New York: Academic Press, 1975.

Cassel, G., Billig, M., and Randall, H. *The Eye Book: A Complete Guide to Eye Disorders and Health*. Baltimore: Johns Hopkins Press Health Book, 1998.

Collins, James. *Your Eyes: An Owner's Guide*. Englewood Cliffs, New Jersey: Prentice Hall, 1995.

Deakins, F., and Grossman, M. *The New Revolution in Eye Care*. Melville, Indiana: America 20/20 Corporation.

Gregory, R. L. *Eye and Brain: The Psychology of Seeing*. London: World University Library, 1969.

Grossman, M., Cooper, R., and N. E. Thing Enterprises. *Magic Eye: How to See 3D*. Kansas City, Missouri: Andrews and McMeel, 1995.

Kavner, R. *Your Child's Vision: A Parent's Guide to Seeing, Growing, and Developing.* New York: Fireside/Simon and Schuster, 1985.

Liberman, J. *Light: Medicine of the Future.* Sante Fe, New Mexico: Bear and Company, 1991.

MacDonald, L. *The Collected Works of Lawrence W. MacDonald*, Vols. 1 and 2. Ira Schwartz and Abraham Shapiro. Santa Ana, California: Optometric Extension Program Foundation, 1993.

Optometric Extension Program Staff Members. *The Primary Visual Abilities Essential to Academic Achievement.* Optometric Extension Program Foundation, 1964, 57.

Chapter 2

Cool, S. "What the Cat's Brain Tells the Vision Therapist," Vol. 34, no. 3, *Optometric Extension Program Vision Therapist*, 1992, 38–101.

Elias, J., and Ketcham, K. *The Five Elements of Self-Healing.* New York: Harmony Books, 1998.

Kohler, L. "Experiments with Goggles." *Scientific American*, 1962, 206: 62–72.

Ross, J. *Acupuncture Point Combinations: The Key to Clinical Success.* New York: Churchill Livingstone, 1995, 21–35, 420.

Severston, E. "Visual Perception," Vol. 38, no. 2, *Optometric Extension Program*, 1996.

Zanjonc, A. *Catching the Light: The Entwined History of Light and Mind.* New York: Bantam, 1993, 1–2.

Chapter 3

Elias, J., and Ketcham, K. *The Five Elements of Self-Healing.* New York: Harmony Books, 1998.

Grossman, M., and Swartwout, G. *Natural Eye Care: An Encyclopedia.* New Canaan, Connecticut: Keats Publishing, 1999.

Huxley, A. *The Art of Seeing.* Seattle: Montana Books, 1975.

Kaptchuk, T. *The Web That Has No Weaver.* New York: Congdon and Weed, 1983.

Lowen, A. *The Betrayal of the Body.* London: Collier MacMillan, 1967.

Chapter 4

Grossman, M., Cooper, R., and N. E. Thing Enterprises. *Magic Eye: How to See 3D*. Kansas City, Missouri: Andrews and McMeel, 1995.

Grossman, M., and Swartwout, G. *Natural Eye Care: An Encyclopedia*. New Canaan, Connecticut: Keats Publishing, 1999.

Quackenbush, T. *Relearning to See*. Berkeley, California: North Atlantic Books, 1997.

Scheiman, M. *Understanding and Managing Vision Deficits: A Guide for Occupational Therapists*. Thorofare, New Jersey: Slack Inc., 1997.

Chapter 5

Berne, S. *Creating Your Personal Vision*. Santa Fe, New Mexico: Color Stone Press, 1994.

Goodrich, J. *Natural Vision Improvement*. Berkeley, California: Celestial Arts, 1985.

Grossman, M., Cooper, R., and N. E. Thing Enterprises. *Magic Eye: How to See 3D*. Kansas City, Missouri: Andrews and McMeel, 1995.

Kaplan, R. M. *Seeing Without Glasses*. Hillsboro, Oregon: Beyond Words, 1994.

Kavner, R., and Dusky, L. *Total Vision*. Millwood, New York: Kavner Books, 1978.

Ross, J. *Acupuncture Point Combinations: The Key to Clinical Success*. New York: Churchill Livingstone, 1995.

Chapter 6

Anshel, J. *Smart Medicine for Your Eyes*. Garden City Park, New York: Avery Publishing, 1999.

Burton Goldberg Group, ed. *Alternative Medicine*. Fife, Washington: Future Medicine Publishers, 1994.

Elias, J., and Masline, R. *Healing Herbal Remedies*. New York: Dell Publishing, 1995.

Lowen, A. *The Betrayal of the Body*. London: Collier MacMillan, 1967.

Quackenbush, T. *Relearning to See*. Berkeley, California: North Atlantic Books, 1997.

Scheiman, M. *Understanding and Managing Vision Deficits: A Guide for Occupational Therapists*. Thorofare, New Jersey: Slack Inc., 1997.

Trachtman, J. N. *The Etiology of Vision Disorders: A Neuroscience Model*. Santa Ana, California: Optometric Extension Program Foundation, 1990.

Trachtman, J. N. Biofeedback of Accommodation Training. Paper presented at the American Academy of Optometry Convention. Philadelphia, 1982.

Trachtman, J. N. Myopia Reduction Using Biofeedback of Accommodation: Summary Results of 100 Patients. Paper presented at the National Eye Research Foundation. Hamilton, Bermuda, 1985.

Chapter 7

Bates, W. H. *The Bates Method for Better Eyesight Without Glasses*. New York: Jove/Harcourt Brace Jovanovich, 1978.

Forrest, E. B. *Visual Imagery: An Optometric Approach*. Santa Ana, California: Optometric Extension Program, 1981.

MacDonald, L. *The Collected Works of Lawrence W. MacDonald*, Vols. 1 and 2. Ira Schwartz and Abraham Shapiro. Santa Ana, California: Optometric Extension Program Foundation, 1993.

Quackenbush, T. *Relearning to See*. Berkeley, California: North Atlantic Books, 1997, 25, 101–103, 477.

Seiderman, A. S., and Marcus, S. E. *20/20 Is Not Enough: The New World of Vision*. New York: Ballantine Books, 1989.

Valenti, C. *Essays on Vision: King of Manifest*. Optometric Extension Program Curriculum II, 1990, 65–84.

Chapter 8

Berne, S. *Creating Your Personal Vision*. Santa Fe, New Mexico: Color Stone Press, 1994.

Grossman, M., and Sweet, C. Monocular Syntonics. Lecture at Annual College of Syntonics Meeting. Ellenville, New York, 1994.

Kaplan, R. M. *The Power Behind Your Eyes.* Rochester, Vermont: Inner Traditions, 1995.

Kaplan, R. M. *Seeing Without Glasses.* Hillsboro, Oregon: Beyond Words, 1994.

Chapter 9

Bates, W. H. *The Bates Method for Better Eyesight Without Glasses.* New York: Jove/Harcourt Brace Jovanovich, 1978.

Grossman, M., Cooper, R., and N. E. Thing Enterprises. *Magic Eye: How to See 3D.* Kansas City, Missouri: Andrews and McMeel, 1995.

MacDonald, L. *The Collected Works of Lawrence W. MacDonald,* Vols. 1 and 2. Ira Schwartz and Abraham Shapiro. Santa Ana, California: Optometric Extension Program Foundation, 1993.

Chapter 10

Bates, W. H. *The Bates Method for Better Eyesight Without Glasses.* New York: Jove/Harcourt Brace Jovanovich, 1978.

Beresford, S., et al. *Improve Your Vision Without Glasses or Contact Lenses.* New York: Simon and Schuster, 1996.

MacDonald, L. *The Collected Works of Lawrence W. MacDonald,* Vols. 1 and 2. Ira Schwartz and Abraham Shapiro. Santa Ana, California: Optometric Extension Program Foundation, 1993.

Swartwout, B. *Optometric Vision Therapy Manual.* Santa Ana, California: Optometric Extension Program Foundation, 1991.

Chapter 11

MacDonald, L. *The Collected Works of Lawrence W. MacDonald,* Vols. 1 and 2. Ira Schwartz and Abraham Shapiro. Santa Ana, California: Optometric Extension Program Foundation, 1993.

Optometric Extension Program. *Vision Therapy: Visual Thinking for Problem Solving,* Vol. 38, no. 3. Santa Ana, California: Optometric Extension Program, 1997.

Swartwout, B. *Optometric Vision Therapy Manual.* Santa Ana, California: Optometric Extension Program Foundation, 1991.

Chapter 12

Berne, S. *Creating Your Personal Vision*. Santa Fe, New Mexico: Color Stone Press, 1994.

Kaplan, R. M. *Seeing Without Glasses*. Hillsboro, Oregon: Beyond Words, 1994.

MacDonald, L. *The Collected Works of Lawrence W. MacDonald*, Vols. 1 and 2. Ira Schwartz and Abraham Shapiro. Santa Ana, California: Optometric Extension Program Foundation, 1993.

Samuels, M., and Samuels, N. *Seeing with the Mind's Eye*. New York: Random House, 1975.

Swartwout, B. *Optometric Vision Therapy Manual*. Santa Ana, California: Optometric Extension Program Foundation, 1991.

Glossary

accommodation: The ability to change the focus of the eye so that objects at different distances can be seen clearly.

acupuncture: A form of medicine that uses fine needles on specific points of the body to achieve balance in a person's energy.

amblyopia (lazy eye): A decrease in sight of one eye that is not correctable with glasses. It happens when the brain ignores some of the information coming from that eye.

anisometropia: When each eye has different refractive powers.

anterior chamber: The space between the cornea and the lens that is filled with a watery fluid called the aqueous humor.

aqueous humor: The clear watery fluid that fills the eye's anterior chamber. Its primary function is to provide nutrients to the cornea and lens and to remove waste. Too much aqueous humor may cause glaucoma.

astigmatism: A condition caused by an irregularity in the shape of the cornea (and/or lens) of the eye that makes the cornea more football-shaped than round.

Bates method: A system of eye exercises originated by William Bates, M.D., to help improve eyesight.

bifocal lens: A lens that has two parts, usually the top for distance vision and the bottom for near vision.

binocular vision: The brain's ability to combine images from each eye into one image.

biofeedback training: A technique for learning self-control over bodily functions.

cataract: A condition where the lens of the eye begins to become opaque.

ciliary muscle: The muscle attached to the lens that is responsible for the skill of accommodation (focusing).

concave lens: A lens whose thinnest portion is in the center; usually used for nearsightedness.

cones: The light-sensitive cells in the retina responsible for detail sight and color vision.

conjunctiva: A thin, clear membrane that covers and protects the white portion of the eye (sclera) and the inner portion of the eyelid.

contact lenses: The transparent plastic lenses worn over the corneas of the eyes to correct vision problems.

convergence: The simultaneous turning in of both eyes that occurs when viewing an approaching object.

convergence excess: When the eyes turn inward toward each other when focusing on a near object.

convergence insufficiency: When the eyes are unable to converge (move toward each other) when looking at a near object.

convex lens: A lens whose thickest portion is in the center; usually used for farsightedness.

cornea: The transparent, blood-free tissue covering the central front of the eye (over the pupil, iris, and aqueous humor) where initial refraction or bending of light rays occurs as light enters the eye.

cover test: A test of the eyes' alignment in which each eye is covered and then uncovered while their movement is observed.

cylinder lens: A lens in which at least one of the surfaces is nonspherical; used for astigmatism.

depth perception: The ability to judge distances by interpreting size, shape, shadows, and overlapping images.

developmental optometry: A branch of optometry that deals with the visual development of children.

diopter: The unit of measurement that describes the power of a lens.

divergence: The simultaneous turning out of both eyes when viewing an object that is moving away from the eyes.

dominant eye: The eye that a person prefers to use to "sight" objects.

esophoria: The muscle alignment of the two eyes when they are turning in toward each other.

esotropia: The inward deviation of the eyes toward each other, better known as crossed eyes.

exophoria: The tendency of the eyes to diverge, or turn away from each other.

exotropia: The outward deviation of the eyes from each other.

extraocular muscles: The muscles attached to the outside of the eyeball, which control eye movements. Each eye has six muscles.

eyeball: The sense organ of the body that receives light and begins processing it into perceived images. Approximately one inch in diameter, the eyeball functions like a camera.

farsightedness (hyperopia): When light passes through the eye and it focuses behind the retina. Those who are farsighted usually have more difficulty with close vision than distance vision.

fixation: The ability of the eyes to attend to a stationary target.

fovea: A tiny depression in the center of the retina's macula region where sight is best and where more cones are found.

fusion: The merging of the images from each eye into a single visual image.

glaucoma: An eye disease that occurs when the eye pressure affects the optic nerve; may cause a decrease in visual field.

homeopathy: Potenized (serial dilution and agitation) remedies prescribed according to similarity of symptoms.

hypertropia: When one eye is higher than the other.

iris: The colored part of the eye.

lens: The part of the eye responsible for changing its shape so light can focus on the retina.

macula: The part of the retina where detailed vision occurs.

monocular vision: Using only one eye.

nearsightedness (myopia): The inability of the eyes to see objects at a distance.

ophthalmoscope: An instrument used to see the back of the eye.

optic nerve: The bundle of nerve fibers that connect the eye to the brain.

phoropter: An instrument containing millions of lens combinations used to help determine a person's prescription; also known as a refractor.

photophobia: Light sensitivity.

presbyopia: The natural decrease of the eye's ability to focus at near distance. It occurs with age and is due to a gradual stiffening of the lens of the eye.

prism lens: A lens that bends light in a specific direction; usually used for muscle problems.

progressive lens: A lens with different prescriptions from the center of the lens to the bottom.

pupil: The black hole in the center of the iris through which light enters the eye.

pursuit eye movements: The ability of the eyes to follow a moving target.

refraction: The determination of lens powers necessary to correct specific amounts of myopia, hyperopia, astigmatism, or presbyopia.

refractive error: Measures the amount of prescription needed so images will appear clearly on the retina.

retina: The light-sensitive tissue in the back of the eye.

retinoscope: An instrument used to measure the bending of light into a person's eyes. It gives an approximation of his or her prescription for glasses.

rods: The light-sensitive cells in the retina that respond to light and dark, movement, and shapes but not to colors.

saccadic eye movements: The eyes' movement from one target to another.

sclera: The white outer covering of the eye.

sight: The eyes' ability to discriminate different objects.

Snellen fraction: A score written as a fraction that is given to each eye; 20/20 is considered ideal. This means that the eye sees at a distance of twenty feet what it should ideally see at twenty feet. As an example, when an eye can see at only twenty feet what it should see at forty feet, it scores 20/40.

strabismus: When the two eyes do not work properly together. The eye may turn in, out, or up.

tonometer: An instrument used to measure the pressure of the fluid contents of the eyeball.

20/20: The normal visual acuity as measured by the use of a wall chart and the Snellen fraction.

vision: A person's ability to interpret and gain meaning from what he or she sees.

visual acuity: The clarity of eyesight.

visual field: The extent of physical space visible to an eye in a given position. Its average extent is sixty-five degrees upward, seventy-five degrees downward, sixty degrees inward, and ninety-five degrees outward.

visual pathway: The route the nerve impulses take from the retina to the optic nerve to the brain.

visual spectrum: The colors visible to the human eye: red, orange, yellow, green, blue, indigo, and violet.

vitreous humor: The fluid located between the lens of the eye and the retina that helps maintain the eye's shape.

Resources

F or more information about vision, contact the following organizations.

General Vision Resources

American Academy of Ophthalmology
Public Information Program
P.O. Box 7424
San Francisco, CA 94210-7424
(415) 561-8500
E-mail: ips@aao.org
Brochures and fact sheets on eye conditions and visual impairment.

American Optometric Association
243 North Lindbergh Boulevard
St. Louis, MO 63141
(800) 365-2219
National office for professional optometry. Patient information materials on vision conditions are available.

____ 1ore Academy for Behavioral Optometry
110 Old Padonia Road
Timonium, MD 21093
(410) 561-3791
Website: www.babousa.org

College of Optometrists in Vision Development (COVD)
353 H. Street, Suite C
Chula Vista, CA 92010
(619) 425-6191
For referrals to a behavioral optometrist.

Optometric Extension Program Foundation, Inc.
2912 South Daimler Street
Santa Ana, CA 92705
(949) 250-8070
For referrals to a behavioral optometrist. The foundation also has books and materials dedicated to behavioral vision care.

Vision Improvement Resources

The following resources offer books, products, and programs for natural vision improvement.

Beyond 20/20 Vision
Roberto Michael Kaplan, O.D.
RR 2, S26C39
Gibson, British Columbia
VON1VO Canada
(604) 888-0608
Website: www.integratedvisiontherapy.com

Cambridge Institute for Better Vision
Martin Sussman
65 Wenham Road
Topsfield, MA 01938
(800) 372-3937

Institute of Visual Healing
Grace Halloran, Ph.D.
655 Lewelling Boulevard, #214
San Leandro, CA 94579
(510) 357-0477

Universal Light Technologies (ULT)
Jacob Liberman, O.D., Ph.D.
P.O. Box 520
Carbondale, CO 81623
(800) 815-4448
E-mail: infor@jacobliberman.com

Vision Works, Inc.
Marc Grossman, O.D., L.Ac.
3 Paradise Lane
New Paltz, New York 12561
(888) 735-8475
(212) 410-0991
Website: www.visionworksusa.com

Recommended Reading

Alternative Medicine

Anshel, J. *Smart Medicine for Your Eyes*. New York: Avery Publishing, 1999.

Burton Goldberg Group, ed. *Alternative Medicine*. Fife, Washington: Future Medicine Publishers, Inc., 1994.

Gimbel, T. *Form, Sound, Colour, and Healing*. Essex, England: The C. W. Daniel Company, 1987.

Grossman, M., and Swartwout, G. *Natural Eye Care: An Encyclopedia*. New Canaan, Connecticut: Keats Publishing, 1999.

Hahnemann, S. *The Organon of the Medical Art*. Redmond, Washington: Birdcage Books, 1997.

McCabe, V. *Homeopathy, Healing, and You*. New York: St. Martins Press, 1997.

McCabe, V. *Practical Homeopathy*. New York: St. Martins Press, 2000.

Richmond, L. *The Vision of Homeopathy: The Mental Symptoms of Vision Syndromes*. Self-published, 1999.

Schwarz, J. *Human Energy Systems*. New York: EP Dutton, 1980.

Art

Edwards, B. *Drawing on the Artist Within*. New York: Simon and Schuster, 1986.

Franck, F. *The Zen of Seeing*. New York: Vintage Books, 1973.

Behavioral Vision Care Philosophy

Dawkins, H., Edelman, E., and Forkiotis, C. *Suddenly Successful: How Behavioral Optometry Helps You Overcome Learning, Health, and Behavior Problems.* Santa Ana, California: Optometric Extension Program Foundation, 1988.

Forrest, E. B. *The Psychobiology of Visual Behavior.* Series 1, 41, (4) Santa Ana, California: Optometric Extension Program Foundation, 1969.

Forrest, E. B. *Stress and Vision.* Santa Ana, California: Optometric Extension Program Foundation, 1988.

Forrest, E. B. *Visual Imagery: An Optometric Approach.* Santa Ana, California: Optometric Extension Program, 1981.

Getman, G. N. *How to Develop Your Child's Intelligence.* Luverne, Minnesota: The Announcer Press, 1958.

Gottlieb, R. "Neuropsychology of Myopia," *Journal of Optometric Vision Development,* Vol. 13, no. 1 (March 1982): 9.

Huxley, A. *The Art of Seeing.* Seattle: Montana Books, 1975.

Jones, B. *Visual Behavior.* Cincinnati: Lockwood Press, 1990.

Kaplan, R. M. *Conscious Seeing.* Hillsboro, Oregon: Beyond Words, 2001.

Kaplan, R. M. *The Power Behind Your Eyes.* Rochester, Vermont: Inner Traditions, 1995.

Kavner, R. *Your Child's Vision: A Parent's Guide to Seeing, Growing, and Developing.* New York: Fireside/Simon and Schuster, 1985.

Kavner, R., and Dusky, L. *Total Vision.* Millwood, New York: Kavner Books, 1978.

Kelly, C. "Psychological Factors in Myopia," *Journal of the American Optometric Association* 33 (6): 1962.

Liberman, J. *Light: Medicine of the Future.* Santa Fe, New Mexico: Bear and Company, 1991.

Liberman, J. *Take Off Your Glasses and See: How to Heal Your Eyesight and Expand Your Insight.* New York: Crown Publishers, 1995.

MacDonald, L. *The Collected Works of Lawrence W. MacDonald,* Vols. 1 and 2. Ira Schwartz and Abraham Shapiro. Santa Ana, California: Optometric Extension Program Foundation, 1993.

Optometric Extension Program Staff Members. *The Primary Visual Abilities Essential to Academic Achievement.* Santa Ana, California: Optometric Extension Program Foundation, 1964.

Orfield, A. "Seeing Space: Undergoing Brain Reprogramming to Reduce Myopia," *Journal of Behavioral Optometry* 5 (5): 123–131.

Scheiman, M. *Understanding and Managing Vision Deficits: A Guide for Occupational Therapists.* Thorofare, New Jersey: Slack Inc., 1997.

Schneider, M. *Self-Healing: My Life and Vision.* New York: Arkana/Viking Penguin, 1987.

Seiderman, A. S., and Marcus, S. E. *20/20 Is Not Enough: The New World of Vision.* New York: Ballantine Books, 1989.

Shankman, A. L. *Skeffington's Emergent-Vision and Psychobehavioral Vision Enhancement,* Vol. 20, *Essays on Vision OEP Curriculum II.* Santa Ana, California: Optometric Extension Program Foundation, 1990.

Shankman, A. L. *Vision Enhancement Training.* Santa Ana, California: Optometric Extension Program Foundation, 1988.

Sutton, A. *Vision, Intelligence, and Creativity.* Santa Ana, California: Optometric Extension Program Foundation, 1988.

Trachtman, J. N. *The Etiology of Vision Disorders: A Neuroscience Model.* Santa Ana, California: Optometric Extension Program Foundation, 1990.

Valenti, C. "Essays on Vision: King of Manifest," *Optometric Extension Program Curriculum II.* Santa Ana, California: Optometric Extension Program Foundation, 1990, 65–84.

Bodywork

Feldenkrais, M. *Awareness Through Movement: Health Exercises for Personal Growth.* New York: Harper & Row, 1972.

Rolf, I. *Rolfing: The Integration of Human Structures.* New York: Harper & Row, 1977.

Sutherland, W. G. "Teachings in the Science of Osteopathy," *Sutherland Cranial Teaching Foundation,* 1990: 230.

Chinese Medicine Philosophy

Elias, J., and Ketcham, K. *The Five Elements of Self-Healing*. New York: Harmony Books, 1998.

Elias, J., and Masline, R. S. *Healing Herbal Remedies*. New York: Dell Publishing, 1995.

Maciocia, G. *The Foundations of Chinese Medicine*. New York: Churchill Livingstone, 1989.

Ross, J. *Acupuncture Point Combinations: The Key to Clinical Success*. New York: Churchill Livingstone, 1995.

Xiangcai, X. *The Encyclopedia of Practical Traditional Chinese Medicine: Ophthalmology*. Beijing, China: Higher Education Press, 1990.

Conventional Vision Care

Cassel, G., Billig, M., and Randall, H. *The Eye Book: A Complete Guide to Eye Disorders and Health*. Baltimore: Johns Hopkins Press Health Book, 1998.

Collins, J. *Your Eyes: An Owner's Guide*. Englewood Cliffs, New Jersey: Prentice Hall, 1995.

Gardner, K. *Eye Movements, Vision, and Behavior*. New York: John Wiley and Sons, 1975.

Hubel, D. *Eye, Brain, and Vision*. New York: Scientific American Library, 1988.

Philosophy

Alexander, F. M. *Resurrection of the Body*. New York: University Books Inc., 1969.

Castaneda, C. *A Separate Reality*. New York: Simon and Schuster, 1971.

Krishnamurti, J. *The Awakening of Intelligence*. New York: Avon Books, 1973.

Ouspensky, P. *The Fourth Way*. New York: Alfred A. Knopf, 1957.

Ouspensky, P. *In Search of the Miraculous*. New York: Harcourt, Brace and World, 1949.

Zukav, G. *The Seat of the Soul*. New York: Simon and Schuster, 1989.

Psychology and Visual Perception

Arnheim, R. *Art and Visual Perception*. Los Angeles: University of California Press, 1954.

Arnheim, R. *Visual Thinking*. London: Faber and Faber, 1969.

Cannon, W. B. *The Wisdom of the Body*. New York: W. W. Norton, 1932.

Carterette, E., and Friedman, M. *Handbook of Perception*. Vol. 5, *Seeing*. New York: Academic Press, 1975.

Dunbar, H. *Emotions and Bodily Changes*. New York: Columbia University Press, 1935.

Gregory, R. L. *Eye and Brain: The Psychology of Seeing*. London: World University Library, 1969.

Kurtz, R. *Hakomi Therapy Manual*. Boulder, Colorado: R. Kurtz, 1985.

Lowen, A. *The Betrayal of the Body*. London: Collier MacMillan, 1967.

Perls, F., Hefferline, R., and Goodman, P. *Gestalt Therapy*. New York: Dell Publishing, 1951.

Riso, D., and Hudson, R. *The Wisdom of the Ennegram*. New York: Bantam Books, 1999.

Samuels, M., and Samuels, N. *Seeing with the Mind's Eye*. New York: Random House, 1975.

Zajone, A. *Catching the Light: The Entwined History of Light and Mind*. New York: Bantam, 1993.

Studies on Vision Therapy

Berman, P. "The Effectiveness of Biofeedback Visual Training as a Viable Method of Treatment and Reduction of Myopia," *Journal of Optometric Vision Development* 16 (1985): 17–21.

Birnbaum, M. "Holistic Aspects of Visual Style: A Hemispheric Model with Implications for Vision Therapy," *Journal of the American Optometric Association* 49 (10) (1978): 1133–1141.

Cohen, B. et al. "Do Hyperactive Children Have Manifestations of Hyperactivity of Eye Movements?" *Journal of Optometric Vision Development* 7 (1976): 18.

Cohen, S. I., and Hajoff, J. "Life Events and the Onset of Acute Closed Angle Glaucoma," *Journal of Psychosomatics Research* 16 (1972): 355–361.

Cool, S. "What the Cat's Brain Tells the Vision Therapist's Brain," *Optometric Extension Program Vision Therapist* 34 no. 3 (1992): 38–101.

Cooper, J., and Duckman, R. "Convergence Insufficiency: Incidence, Diagnosis, and Treatment," *Journal of the American Optometric Association* 49 (1978): 673–680.

Croll, M. C., and Croll, L. J. "Emotional Glaucoma," *American Journal of Ophthalmology* 49 (1960): 297–305.

Daum, K. M. "Convergence Insufficiency," *American Journal of Optometry and Physiological Optics* 61 (1984): 16–22.

Fletcher, M., and Silverman, S. "Strabismus: A Study of 1,100 Consecutive Cases," *American Journal of Ophthalmology* 61 no. 25: 86–94.

Goss, D. A., and Winkler, R. L. "Progression of Myopia in Youth: Age of Cessation," *American Journal of Optometry and Physiological Optics* 1983: 651–658.

Grignolo, F. M. et al. "Variations of Intraocular Pressure Induced by Psychological Stress," *Klingishe Monatsblaten Augenheilkd* 170 (1977): 562–569.

Kohler, L. "Experiments with Goggles," *Scientific American* 206 (1962): 62–72.

Ludlum, W. "Orthoptic Treatment of Strabismus," *American Journal of Optometry and Archives of the American Academy of Optometry* 42 (November 1965): 647–684.

Moses, R. A., Preston, L., and Wette, R. "Horizontal Gaze Position Effect on Intraocular Pressure," *Investigative Ophthalmology* 22 (1982): 551–53.

Pantano, R. "Orthoptic Treatment of Convergence Insufficiency: A Two-Year Follow-Up Report," *American Orthoptic Journal* 32 (1982): 73–80.

Passo, M. S. et al. "Exercise Training Reduces Intraocular Pressure Among Subjects Suspected of Having Glaucoma," *Archives of Ophthalmology* 109 (1991): 1096–98.

"Personalities Differ in Visual Systems," *Brain/Mind Bulletin* October 3, 1983.

Rosner, M., and Belkin, M. "Intelligence, Education, and Myopia in Males," *Archives of Ophthalmology* 105 (1987): 1508–1511.

"School Anxiety May Be Major Cause of Myopia," *Brain/Mind Bulletin* 7 no. 17.

Sherman, A. "Myopia Can Be Prevented, Controlled, or Eliminated," *Journal of Behavioral Optometry* 4 (1993): 16.

Trachtman, J. N. "Biofeedback of Accommodation to Reduce Myopia—A Review," *American Journal of Optometry and Physiological Optics* 64 (8): 639–643.

Trachtman, J. N. Biofeedback of Accommodation Training. Paper presented at the American Academy of Optometry Convention. Philadelphia, 1982.

Trachtman, J. N. Myopia Reduction Using Biofeedback of Accommodation: Summary Results of 100 Patients. Paper presented at the National Eye Research Foundation. Hamilton, Bermuda, 1985.

Trachtman, J. N., and Giambalvo, V. "The Baltimore Myopia Study 40 Years Later." *Journal of Behavioral Optometry* 1991 2: 47–50.

Trachtman, J. N., Giambalvo, V., and Feldman, V. "Biofeedback of Accommodation to Reduce Functional Myopia," *Biofeedback Self-Regulation* 1981, 6 (4): 547–562.

"Vision Training Provides Window to Brain Change," *Brain/Mind Bulletin* 7 no. 17.

Von Senden, M. *Space and Sight: The Perception of Space and Shape in the Congenitally Blind Before and After Operation.* trans. Peter Heath. Glencoe, Illinois: The Free Press, 1960.

Wiggins, N., and Daum, K. "Visual Discomfort and Astigmatic Refractive Errors in VDT Use," *Journal of the American Optometric Association* 68 (1991): 680–684.

Young, F. A. "The Effect of Restricted Visual Space on the Refractive Error of the Young Monkey Eye," *Investigative Ophthalmology* 2 (1963): 571–577.

Young, F. A. et al. "The Transmission of Refractive Errors Within Eskimo Families," *Archives of the American Academy of Optometry* 49 (1969): 676–685.

Zeki, S. "The Visual Image in Mind and Brain," *Scientific American.* 1992, 267 (3): 69–76.

Vision Therapy and Eye Exercises

Bates, W. H. *The Bates Method for Better Eyesight Without Glasses.* New York: Jove/Harcourt Brace Jovanovich, 1978.

Beresford, S. et al. *Improve Your Vision Without Glasses or Contact Lenses.* New York: Simon and Schuster, 1996.

Berne, S. *Creating Your Personal Vision.* Santa Fe, New Mexico: Color Stone Press, 1994.

Corbett, M. *Help Yourself to Better Sight.* North Hollywood, California: Wilshire Book Co., 1949.

Friedman, E., with Lilow, K. *Dr. Friedman's Vision Training Program.* New York: Bantam, 1983.

Goodrich, J. *Natural Vision Improvement.* Berkeley, California: Celestial Arts, 1985.

Griffin, J. *Binocular Anomalies Procedures for Vision Therapy.* Chicago: Professional Press, 1976.

Grossman, M., Cooper, R., and N. E. Thing Enterprises. *Magic Eye: How to See 3D.* Kansas City, Missouri: Andrews and McMeel, 1995.

Harris, P. *Myopia Control in China.* Santa Ana, California: Optometric Extension Program Foundation, 1981.

Kaplan, R. M. *Seeing Without Glasses.* Hillsboro, Oregon: Beyond Words, 1994.

Kraskin, Robert A. *You Can Improve Your Vision.* Garden City, New York: Doubleday and Company Inc., 1968.

Leviton, R. *Seven Steps to Better Vision.* Brookline, Massachusetts: East/West Natural Health Books, 1992.

Marston, W. "Visual Vignette: Eyes Are Mirrors of the Mind," *Journal of Optometric Vision Development,* Vol. 24, no. 1, Spring 1993.

Nelson, J. Visual Acuity in Myopia. Dissertation, College of Optometry, Pacific University.

Quackenbush, T. *Relearning to See.* Berkeley, California: North Atlantic Books, 1997.

Rosannes-Berret, M. *Do You Really Need Glasses?* Barrytown, New York: Station Hill Press, 1990.

Rotte, J., and Yamamoto, K. *Vision: A Holistic Guide to Healing the Eyesight*. New York: Japan Publications, 1986.

Scholl, L. *Visionetics: The Holistic Way to Better Eyesight*. Garden City, New York: Doubleday, 1978.

Selby, J. *The Visual Handbook: The Complete Guide to Seeing More Clearly*. Dorset, England: Element Books, 1987.

Sussman, M. *Program for Better Vision*. Cambridge, Massachusetts: Cambridge Institute for Better Vision, 1985.

Swartwout, B. *Optometric Vision Therapy*. Santa Ana, California: Optometric Extension Program Foundation, 1991.

Index

Myopia
Convergence
Excess